Meditation

Explore Techniques for Practicing Mindfulness

(Science-influenced Approach to Self Care Through Breathwork & Meditation)

Arturo McLean

Published By **Jordan Levy**

Arturo McLean

All Rights Reserved

Meditation: Explore Techniques for Practicing Mindfulness (Science-influenced Approach to Self Care Through Breathwork & Meditation)

ISBN 978-1-7777786-9-9

No part of this guidebook shall be reproduced in any form without permission in writing from the publisher except in the case of brief quotations embodied in critical articles or reviews.

Legal & Disclaimer

The information contained in this book is not designed to replace or take the place of any form of medicine or professional medical advice. The information in this book has been provided for educational & entertainment purposes only.

The information contained in this book has been compiled from sources deemed reliable, and it is accurate to the best of the Author's knowledge; however, the Author cannot guarantee its accuracy and validity and cannot be held liable for any errors or omissions. Changes are periodically made to this book. You must consult your doctor or get professional medical advice before using any of the suggested remedies, techniques, or information in this book.

Upon using the information contained in this book, you agree to hold harmless the Author from and against any damages, costs, and expenses, including any legal fees potentially resulting from the application of any of the information provided by this guide. This disclaimer applies to any damages or injury caused by the use and application, whether directly or indirectly, of any advice or information presented, whether for breach of contract, tort, negligence, personal injury, criminal intent, or under any other cause of action.

You agree to accept all risks of using the information presented inside this book. You need to consult a professional medical practitioner in order to ensure you are both able and healthy enough to participate in this program.

Table Of Contents

Chapter 1: How Do You Sit And How To Position Your Body 1

Chapter 2: The Voice That Is Behind The Voice 11

Chapter 3: How Do You Breathe? 21

Chapter 4: Grounding & Resourcing 42

Chapter 5: The Wall Gazing Meditation . 54

Chapter 6: What Is Mindfulness Meditation? 74

Chapter 7: Breathing Techniques 83

Chapter 8: Emotions 91

Chapter 9: Silence 101

Chapter 10: Pain 112

Chapter 11: Loving-Kindness 123

Chapter 12: The Benefits That Come From Mindfulness And Meditation 140

Chapter 13: Understanding The Mind-Body Connection 143

Chapter 14: How To Practice Loving-Kindness Meditation 150

Chapter 15: How To Practice Walking Meditation 156

Chapter 16: How To Practice Mindful Movement 164

Chapter 17: Mindfulness And Meditation For Anxiety And Depression 172

Chapter 18: Mindfulness And Meditation For Better Relationships 182

Chapter 1: How Do You Sit And How To Position Your Body

Meditation can be performed in many places; however some have more benefits for relaxation and focus in comparison to other positions. Find the best position for you is an exercise of trying out various positions and selecting the one you enjoy. So long as you have your spine straight you'll be in good shape.

Here are some suggestions for getting the ideal posture for meditation.

1. Choose a stable and comfortable seat or cushion. It is essential when you use the chair that it is comfortable and straight with your back straight and your feet straight on the ground. Don't lean to far, since this could cause sleepiness or discomfort.

2. Find a posture that permits you to keep a good posture. Proper posture means keeping your spine straight, and your

shoulders in a relaxed position, keeping your head at a level position and your chin tucked slightly.

3. Certain people prefer sitting in a crossed-legged sitting position on a cushion some prefer a seat that has backrest. Many argue against using the backrest for support of your back, however I've never had a problem regarding back support. Most important is finding a place which allows you to unwind and remain conscious at the same.

4. Be sure to have plenty of space for stretching your arms and legs. Being in a cramped, overcrowded spaces can make you feel uncomfortable and uncomfortable.

5. A bed positioned on top of yours can be effective, but it's not advised, as it is associated with sleep and generally challenging to remain awake and active. It can be useful for exercises in visualization that can be done while lying down.

While more intense meditation techniques can force people to become comfortable discomfort, such as being on solid surfaces for prolonged periods in time. I do not believe that this approach is beneficial to the vast majority of us. I'd recommend sitting in a manner which allows you to remain as alert and comfortable. If you're doing it with your legs crossed or on a stool so long as you are able to keep your spine and back straight then you're in good shape.

When you sit in certain positions particularly cross-legged ones there is the possibility of having your legs go in a state of numbness during your meditation. If you notice numbness, or pain within your legs when being cross-legged in meditation you should alter your posture and position towards a more relaxed position. The constant numbness or discomfort could create distractions and cause you to be unable to concentrate in your meditation.

Relaxation

When you begin your meditation session before you begin your meditation practice, you must bring your entire body into the state of relaxation. The key is to release tension that is in your muscles. When you ease every muscle you have it will be apparent that your mind is also relaxed.

It's helpful to contract muscles prior to relaxing them. In this way, you'll be capable of identifying those muscles that you're focusing on. You can also sense the difference as you ease that tension. You don't need to go overboard with your tension. Do it until an extent that you feel tension.

Start with the upper part of your head, tighten your muscles and relax every muscle throughout your body. You will work towards your toes. When you're done then take a deep breath in, and exhale at a slow pace. There are some areas, such as the head's top aren't muscles that could be stretched. If this is the case, think of tensing the body. You will get the same benefits.

Make your forehead wrinkle and hold for a few seconds then release.

Close your eyes and keep it for a couple of seconds after which you can relax.

Keep your jaw closed and keep it for a short time, then let your jaw relax.

Tensify the muscles of your shoulders and neck, relax them and let them fall.

Make sure you tighten your fists, and then the muscles that are in your hands and arms, after which you can let them loose and let them go limp.

Inhale deeply and hold for a few seconds. Exhale and breathe out.

Intensify your abdominal muscles Then allow them to go.

Relax your back, and arch it for a few seconds after which you can relax.

Tensify the muscles of your back and hips. after which you release them and let them loose.

Toes should be pointed and you must tense your muscles around your feet and legs, after which you release them and let them relax.

Once you are on your toes then take several deep breaths, and concentrate on the feeling of your breath flowing in the body and then out. Let your mind relax and be focused on the current moment.

This will prepare you to meditate.

The itching, snoring and swallowing

Once you are in your routine you might be distracted by a few things immediately. The first is you could feel the need to take a swallow. It's okay, even when it appears excessive to the person who is eating it. This could be a subconscious method of distraction, but so it does not stop the flow, it typically reverses the process.

Keep in mind that what you consume and drinks can affect the saliva reaction. Drinking water, citrus or food that demand a lot of chewing can cause this to increase so pay attention to the foods you consume prior to you begin your meditation.

Another frequent distraction is itching sensations. There are many sources that say that it's best to just let the itching sensation to occur and it'll go away within just a couple of seconds. However, for me, that's not an option. If I do my best to avoid it however, the more intense I think it is to become, and I scratch whenever I have to and then keep practicing. Choose the method that works for you.

Where is my tongue going?

I have found that if you keep the tongue in the top of your mouth, with the tips touching to the rear of your teeth is the most optimal way to go.

It promotes relaxation of the face and jaw and can relax the body and mind. It helps focus and can aid in sharpening the focus of your mind and lessen the distraction of thoughts.

Also, it regulates breath by it encourages slow, deep and even deep breaths.

When you apply your tongue's touch to the surface of the mouth activates the vagus nerve. It is a nerve that connects the brain to the digestive system, encouraging relaxation as well as reducing anxiety.

How long should you meditate?

The benefits you will reap from continuous practice of meditation whether for just a few minutes or one hour. It is evident that the longer you exercise, the more advantages. Based on my own observation, I'm in the zone about 20 minutes. The result is an alteration in my brainwave activity, which takes me to a higher level. The experience can feel as if I'm asleep but remaining conscious simultaneously.

Be aware that this does not often occur and neither is it something to be feared. Your experience with meditation may depend upon a myriad of variables that cannot be completely controlled by you. This is merely a interval that I've enjoyed my experience. It is possible that your experience will be different.

Are I making a mistake?

There's nothing wrong with the practice of meditation. It helps you grow and improve as you progress. There's no destination that you must be, but the place you are currently. Some practices can yield better performance, however after you've learned some fundamentals and you'll be able to discover more by putting them into repetition.

How do we deal with too many thoughts?

While it is wonderful to experience absolutely no thoughts in your training, it is not the ideal. Thoughts are bound to happen. It's common. You'll probably most of the time think more than you would like. This "monkey brain" is not an automatic process that decides to shut down. It's just a matter of time and constant repetition

One of the first points you need to draw concerning your thoughts is the fact the fact that you're not the thoughts you think of and the thoughts you think of aren't yours. They're separate even when they're sometimes inseparable. Your real core, isn't the thought part of your. The calm is behind your thinking. Imagine it as the ocean. While the surface may be undergoing a huge storm, under the surface it is all peaceful. If you dig deep enough there's a chance that you don't even see anything whatsoever.

Chapter 2: The Voice That Is Behind The Voice

When you begin to notice your own about thoughts, you'll start to pay attention to the observers of your thoughts too. Much like an onion, there numerous layers of thought. The conscious thoughts that is a thought that says "wow, it's so much quieter in here at this moment" and not conscious of the fact that it was your thought. It's a great location to be. Your mind is calm but the thought hasn't been silenced. This isn't often the case and is okay. Be aware of the thinking of the initial thought will get you one step closer to your part of you which is simply "being".

Another method I employ to calm my mind is to imagine my thoughts. As they pop out, and then I begin to observe words appearing in the distance as if they were a movie screen and then I can create sentences. One of the first steps is to simply observe the thought as if it were the movie, and not let your mind try to be part of the film. The point is to watch, but with no judgement.

In the next step, I'll be able to see those thoughts that come to me as I imagine that sentence or word breaking down. I will see repeatedly the beginning of an idea pattern and let it disintegrate before it's completed. As with everything it is, the more time you spend practicing and practice, the more quickly you can catch the thoughts that are evolving.

We are waiting for the thoughts to come.

It's an effective method which is effective in calming your mind. This is like waiting for a cat on the other side of the mouse hole waiting for it to poke its head so that you can take it in. This time we're thinking about it.

As with waiting for a mouse to click, we'll be waiting on thoughts. For this to happen, you need to mentally consider about yourself "I wonder what I will think next" Then just sit and watch.

There are often times when the person thinking stops and awaits the next thought without conscious that he is also the person who created these ideas. Powerful technique.

The desire to keep things in mind that pop into your the mind

It's a common thing to do during meditation. You may be thinking about things which you've forgotten about or didn't think about for a long time. Sometimes, fresh ideas and solutions could come to mind also. Many of them can be stored away during your work and rediscovered after having completed the practice. Naturally, if there's something that you find too important to be let go of then stop practicing and record it, and then you can return to the practice.

These small insight are a gift that tends to come only from a calm mind. Certain things could be considered crucial, but are actually distraction strategies that are best kept to be put off until when it's time. After some time and practice, you'll recognize the distinction fast.

Focus your inner eyes

While you meditate with your eyes closed It's beneficial to find a spot for your eyes to be focused. What you choose to focus on will affect what kind of experience you experience. The most efficient method is to concentrate on your pineal gland or the one that people refer to as the "third eye". It's the space that lies between the eyebrows that is over the bridge of your nose.

Imagine that your third eye is projected onto a screen that is in the distance. There is no need to look at any thing. Think of it as an oblique glance at a location near the pineal gland without your eyes shut. Most of the time, simply by paying attention to the pineal gland your soft gaze is likely to come easily. Be careful not to focus too hard on your concentration. It should be easy to do everything.

It is a kind of inner focus can help me to go deeper into my practice. It's quite a pleasant experience to feel you are lost in your exercise. It's like everything disappears apart from you and the practice.

If it doesn't happen to you, that's okay and you're not being a fool. In the end, you'll have tiny moments that could take a few minutes. Be aware that trying to create your experience can be the most effective method of not having one. Let your meditation be its job.

Refrain, neutrality, thoughts and quietness

The practice of meditation is mostly of the absence of reaction. Knowing what that actually means could be difficult to master. The brain is a receptive machine. It is aware of what's happening on the outside then compares it to past experiences, and finally has an response. Most of the time it is not your choice to choose the reaction; it's selected by the universe. This happens so rapidly and without efforts and practice the reactions you experience are mostly automated, which means you don't make a decision in the situation.

How many emotions can we experience in day-to-day lives, whether due to current circumstances or thoughts about the past or fears of issues that haven't come to fruition? I'd say a good number.

Meditation is the practice of letting things happen without any reaction. It's an exercise in observing what's going on within the mind, and then let it go instead of focusing on the thought. Because the brain is constantly receptive and in constant motion, a state of calmness and neutrality towards thoughts that arise is a challenge.

Be aware that it's perfectly normal to fail over and over when you try to not react. Your brain can use many techniques in order to trigger your brain to respond. Actually, just two minutes of stillness in mediation can be an advantage. It is a paradox that when not focusing on any goals in your meditation practice it is possible to experience what could be thought to be deeper experiences.

Failure to remain still and inactive isn't a failing it's just a matter of meditation, and you're in no way committing a mistake. Your only failure is to believe that you're not good at meditation and not getting any benefit by it. This is why you should quit. It is possible that your most memorable experiences occur at unplanned occasions. The thing that can trip your nerves is trying to determine the best way to replicate that moment. My only advice I could provide is to simply maintain the habit of relaxing your mind, and to allow the unexpected to happen in your session.

What is the best way to apply non-reaction?

According to my personal experience The first rule of work is to be still. It is about relaxing your body and muscles. When you are still with your body, your thoughts will also follow. There will be moments in which you aren't moving, and also moments when that you did not think. The body might feel an increased vibration while you're in a solitary position. This could be a sign that you're heading towards the right direction.

When you experience sensations, your mind may be screaming "It's working! I'm doing it! " But this can lead to that feeling disappearing. It is at this point that the practice of not reacting to what you experience or think of can be crucial. Another method of explaining the things you wish to accomplish is simply to observe the moment. The goal is not to form an opinion about your experience, but rather let the experience pass by and disappear.

An effective way to think about the non-reaction state is to watch people go by through the window of your bedroom. Consider your thoughts to be just behind the window and only walking through. It's not necessary to get involved with them in any way. At some point, you'll notice the beginnings of thoughts before they've become solidified. If you are able to catch these thoughts early enough they can go back to air. You'll notice the words begin to develop into sentences and then catching the words before they're fully formed and then leaving them to disappear to space.

You've realized that, no matter how hard you work you'll get caught up by your thoughts in the midst of it all. The only thing you have to do is stop yourself, and then shift the focus of your mind towards the breath. It is a way of losing yourself in thoughts and then getting back to breathing. If you're doing this correctly, then you've done it right.

Breathing

Chapter 3: How Do You Breathe?

The breath is the most fundamental method of altering our state of mind, and is a crucial aspect of meditation. It isn't my intention to be an expert in everything breathing, however I will say what's helped myself.

The first thing I do to practice breathing is to become at ease breathing through my nose. Numerous meditation experts recommend breathing through the nose and out with the mouth, but I've discovered that all breathing is done by the nose makes it simpler and more relaxing for me. There's much less thought. If exhaling with the mouth feels more comfortable for you, try it.

After you have mastered simple in-and-out breathing You should learn the art of breathing deeply into your stomach and refrain from shallow breathing in the upper chest. It's more nourishing for your body. The deep stomach breathing technique is fairly effortless once you get grasp of it.

Perineum Breathing

First, you'll be able to understand the position of the perineum which is the place between the anus and the sexual organs. If you think the breath coming from the perineum, you'll begin taking deep belly breaths that we want.

You can place one hands on your stomach while the other is placed on your chest. The stomach should expand with every breath. For me, it is easier to imagine air slapping my chest, and then descending to my lower stomach.

For you to relax in your meditation practice It's helpful to take 5 deep, slow belly breaths. Hold at least 2 seconds for each inhale and exhale. After that, breathe in a normal way, deep into the stomach.

The process should be more natural in time Don't stress excessively about it. The less you need to consider more you can relax.

The sensations that can arise from this exercise could be sensations of warmth or perineum tingling and a greater awareness of bodily sensations and feelings of tranquil and peace.

When practicing during the practice, you must remain focused on the sensations of the perineum. Also, make sure you remain at peace and calm during taking a breath. If you find your mind beginning to wander, just keep your mind focused on breathing and the sensations of the abdomen.

It's also beneficial to maintain your breathing steady and constant, while avoiding over-exaggerated or forceful motions. As time passes and you practice the technique of meditation can assist in quieting your mind, and increase awareness and tranquility.

Be aware that your breath itself isn't moving between the perineum. Instead, your focus should be to direct the breath downwards to your root chakra mental and then letting your breath move deeply into the stomach.

Sensations

When you meditate You may begin experiencing some sensations. It's a great aspect. It typically means that you're getting into a more profound state. Be careful not to pursue the feeling or attempt to manage it.

They'll likely appear with a whimper. As they fade without a trace, you shouldn't believe that you did any wrong. Keep your mind neutral and non-reactive.

Out-breath pause

I've noticed that taking at least a second after taking your exhale before beginning your breath again it, can trigger an energy buzz, or vibration and a deeper sense of relaxation. It can be beneficial to deepen the practice for me.

Be careful not to create a pause that is uncomfortable or rushed or you'll be forced to stop your breathing in order to get a deeper recover breath. It's normal and acceptable for this to occur when you meditate, however you must do all you can to keep the same breathing pattern.

You can feel your energy body's subtle energie let itself breathe

It's a weird feeling when you first experience it. This feels like feeling your breath's intent before taking the breath. As I've experienced, you'll experience the breath sensation inside and the sensation of breathing outside.

I think this is the energy body that is subtle. Like the concept of placing your attention on an area of your body and then noticing a greater sensations in that particular location, you're now experiencing the energy that can make breathing effortless in the absence of it.

Take a moment to breathe in the feeling and observe if it is like it is comfortable for you. If not, you can return to the same rhythm as before and let the gentle flow of energy adapt to the rhythm of your breathing.

How to meditate

While this might be apparent for some, I'm adding this as a reminder of how busy the brain wants to be. It is eager to get things done that are successful and know that things are being done correctly.

Meditation is the antithesis of everything. It's the process of abandoning of the task and doing. It is the process in training your mind to become more aware and focussed. The mind naturally tends to wander and meditate can help reconnect it with the present.

And what can we do when we meditate?

This is contingent on the form of meditation you are doing. As having no thoughts is an extremely difficult process which only lasts for a short time, it is best to provide the brain with things that it can "notice".

It can refer to the breathing out and in breath. Be aware of the sound you hear when breathing, as well as the feeling. It could also become a habit of paying attention and being aware without reacting.

It's not thinking until you assign it an identity or give it an opinion regarding what you're seeing.

Certain meditations require you to visualize images, colors of scenes, sensations or images. This can be more frequent in guided meditations that have usually a predetermined result. This may sound to be an absurdity when you consider that the essence of meditation isn't seeking an outcome, however to rather take in the current moment.

In order to avoid any unnecessary confusion, let's break meditation down into two groups. Focused visualizations and presence. Both of these practices are beneficial to our lives and if you had a goal for meditation, this is the one.

Beginning mind

Beginning to Mind is a term that is often associated with mindfulness or meditation. It is the concept that you approach each the experience from a different view, devoid of any preconceptions or judgements. This is approaching something using an attitude of a novice instead of being an professional.

This allows you to engage in your work by adopting an open and curious mindset, as opposed to one that is fixed or rigid. This allows you to become more in the present and let off any judgements or expectations. This also implies letting go of any criticisms or judgments that you might have regarding your capabilities or performance. Simply approach each exercise in a manner that is open and curious and with no expectations.

It's an ongoing practice of dissolving beliefs, opinions, as well as expectations, and opening up to fresh perspectives. This is the appeal of mindfulness and the practice of meditation. Take note of your feelings and thoughts that come up as you session. Instead of becoming caught with them, or even judging them, just look at them with a non-judgmental approach. This will help you look at your emotions and thoughts in a different way and also get rid of any attachments in them.

Do not compare yourself with others in the course of your exercise. Each person's story is unique so comparing yourself with others may lead to feelings like lack of confidence or discontent. Instead, concentrate upon your own personal experiences and growth, and be proud of your personal achievements.

Closed Eye Meditations

Metabolizing Energy

I was introduced to this practice by Guy Ferdman of Satori Prime It's been a major game change for me. His brother and him Ilan are doing amazing work, and should be checked out.

Here's how to do it.

The aim of this method is to release trapped energetic energy flowing through your body back into motion. The energy that is trapped can come from past experiences, or unhealthy patterns. If left to linger it can cause illnesses, depression and disease. We need to free the energy that is trapped and restore our body back to its normal condition of health and flow.

It is recommended to remain sitting in the or seated position with eyes shut. When you've completed the relaxation phase, calming every muscle, you'll be ready to begin the meditation.

It is important to first feel the energy flow and how you can direct on it. Whatever you concentrate on will increase the flow of energy to that particular area. Take for instance, focusing in your left arm for a minute and you may feel sensation of warmth, buzzing, tingling or a stronger sensation. As you practice, you'll soon notice it in any area of your body you concentrate on. It's the body's subtle energy.

Inhale a few deep belly breaths, both in and out. Inhale through your nostrils and out through your mouth. If you would prefer to breathe out through your mouth, then you may also breath out with the nostrils.

Be aware that anything we are doing in this process is not a burden. The goal isn't to force the energy that you feel to move anyplace. It is simply watching and paying attention to it. It doesn't matter if you experience a shift in energy or not so long as you're only observing, then you are accomplishing this very well.

For this particular meditation focus on the central channel within our body. It is located between your stomach and the head. It is my suggestion that you take a long, slow scan starting inside your stomach all the way towards your heart, and until your neck and the head. The thing we're looking for is the region of your body that appears to feel the strongest. There may be several areas but we'll concentrate on the part that has the greatest feeling.

Be aware that the parts of your body possess a front, back and left and right. Make sure you know the exact position and amount of energy. Do not confuse it with physical injuries right now. While there is a way to bring healing but let's concentrate this practice on the emotional energy that we feel.

If you locate the most energetic and active area, just focus your attention there as you breathe. Remember, you are not trying to cause anything or alter anything. Think of it more as being aware of your body. Simply paying attention will do all it's work on its own. Concentrate on the spot as well as your breath. Inhale deeply into your belly.

When any thoughts or feelings arise, relax and focus on the feeling of your body. If you feel like that it's moving, be aware of it. It's only our job to be observant.

Remain focused on the strongest feeling in the center of your body.

If you are able to do this for more than 20 minutes, it is possible to be able to see over the course of your practice changes are occurring and the body's natural release of the energy that is trapped. Similar to every meditation, stay practice and be patient.

Mantra Meditation

Mantra meditation is a form of meditation where you concentrate your attention on the specific word or sound that is referred to as the mantra. It is chanted, spoken and recited silently within your brain. It is the intention to utilize repetition to relax your mind, and create relaxation and consciousness.

Before you begin, pick the mantra that is most meaningful to your. Below are 10 mantras are commonly used to practice this type of meditation.

Om is a classic Sanskrit mantra, thought to represent the sound that rang out from the universe.

Peace is an easy and soothing word that will create a calm and peaceful atmosphere

The emotion of love can create an emotion of love and affection.

"I am" - this mantra can help bring your attention to the present moment as well as your personal identity

Relax - repeating this sentence can help get rid of tension and negative thought patterns

I am sufficient This mantra is a great way in building self-confidence and confidence in yourself

Repetition of this phrase will help you cultivate an appreciation for gratitude. appreciation

Bliss: focusing on this positive word could provide a feeling of happiness and happiness.

1. Relax into a comfortable sitting posture and do the practice of relaxing your muscles from head to the toe.

2. Inhale deeply while concentrating on the feel of your breath's movement through and out of your body.

3. Start repeating the mantra for yourself, whether out to the world or quietly inside your head.

4. If you find your mind wandering then gently draw your focus towards the mantra.

5. Keep repeating the mantra whatever time you'd like while focusing on the sound as well as the breathing. Make a schedule, so you don't get distracted by the clock ticking.

6. Once you're done then take a few deep breaths before slowly opening your eyes.

The benefits that you can expect to experience through mantra meditation could be the ability to relax, less stress as well as improved concentration as well as a feeling of being connected to the world.

Visualization

The practice of visualization is one of meditation where one focuses his or her attention to a visual image or the collection of pictures or scenes to help create a feeling of peace and ease. It is a method of creating an environment in which one can be free of the stresses and distractions of life and concentrate on their inner thoughts.

Meditation using visual imagery can be utilized to serve a range of reasons that include well-being goals, setting goals, as well as personal development. Many people imagine a certain result or goal to achieve something, for example better health or a prosperous job, while some make use of it to unwind and achieve an inner peace.

Benefits of visualization are an increased sense of control over thoughts and feelings, as well as a peace of mind about the future. Additionally, it can help people in defining their goals and devise strategies to achieve these goals. Visualization can also be a great method for planning and problem solving.

A well-known person who utilized visualization to reach a certain target is Jackie Joyner Kersee, who is a former

American track and field player. Joyner-Kersee has been referred to as among the most outstanding female athletes in history and holds the world record for the heptathlon. It is a event in track and field which consists of seven disciplines.

She would imagine herself the best she could and winning races before events actually took place. The visualizations helped her remain focused and motivated and was a major factor in her accomplishment in her career as an athlete. Indeed, she's stated that visualization was an integral element of her regimen, and she relied on it to get over doubts and fears she was battling about her capabilities.

This is a powerful demonstration of the impact of visualization on a person's ability to accomplish their objectives.

How it is done:

1. Set a goal, or a desire. This can be something simple for example, such as

getting a parking space, or something more significant, such as the search for a new job, or beginning a new friendship.

2. Take a moment to close your eyes, and then breathe deeply. Inhaling, you can imagine that you're filling the body up with positive positive energies. When you exhale, think that you have released your fears or doubts.

3. Make your vision of your goal like it's already accomplished. Picture yourself in the position feeling the emotions and emotions that go with the experience. It is not a good idea to view yourself as if you are observing from afar the objective. It is best to imagine the event as if what you are experiencing through your own eyes. Be as precise as you can be.

4. Keep the image within your head for just a few minutes every daily. This can be done anytime, however it's best to practice it before getting up, after bed or either.

5. In the event that inspiration comes, move forward towards your goal. The power of visualization isn't sufficient to accomplish your goals, however, it can trigger small ideas that you can act upon. Even if your decision doesn't seem to make sense in the moment be sure to trust your intuition and follow the path it takes. The dots will join when the objective was accomplished.

If you keep imagining your goals and doing something about your goal, you will improve the chances of bringing the desired outcome into your daily life. Be flexible and maintain an open mind as events happen by their own means and should not be imposed upon.

If you are constantly focusing about the end goal, it indicates that you're not confident that you can visualize things into your daily everyday life. It should be a way to energize yourself and be fun without causing stress or become another task that you need to tick off your list of things to-do list.

If you are struggling to make things happen, or think "Oh what a mess, I couldn't think about the day before. I've screwed everything up. It's time to fix it." I think you're not getting the message. The process itself involves trusting and surrendering. When visualization causes a lot of anxiety, you should take breaks until the concept of doing it makes sense and enjoyable.

Chapter 4: Grounding & Resourcing

The practice of grounding and resourcing can be an effective practice that will aid in cultivating a profound feeling of harmony, balance and rejuvenating energy. It involves reconnection to the earth's energy and drawing upon the energy of this planet to aid in mental focus, emotional regulation and motivation.

In order to begin the meditation start by finding a peaceful or comfortable space for you to lie or sit. Inhale a few deeply breathing breaths in a slow pace to calm yourself and set the stage for your practice. Next, concentrate your focus on your feet, and visualize roots extending through the heels of your feet down into the ground.

If you can visualize the roots, you will feel being connected to the energies of earth. Feel the energy flow up through the roots, and then through your body and giving you a feeling of stability and grounding. Be aware of the energies that comes from earth nurturing and sustaining you. Then let yourself relax to this sensation of security and security.

Think of the energy of earth flowing upwards through your roots in your body, filling you with life and energy. Be open to any ideas and insights or ideas that might arise. Be awed by the body's wisdom and the energy of earth that will guide you to higher clarity, focus and intuition.

The practice is either short or as long as you consider essential. Just 5 minutes of practice can make a an impact positive on the day. When we connect with the energy of the earth, we are able to develop a sense of grounding and enthusiasm that helps people navigate the challenges of life in a more relaxed and resilient manner.

Earthing

A great method to get grounded is to do a simple method, which is also known as earthing. It's a method of linking your body with the natural energy of the earth through physical contact.

An easy and simple technique to become grounded is by standing barefoot on grass. It has plenty of mental and physical health benefits, such as allowing your body to absorb electrons that are free that come from the earth. This helps neutralize free radicals, and help lessen inflammation.

This can help to improve circulation, balance hormones and boost immune system function.

Deep void meditation

The practice will allow you to go deep within your own self. The meditation masters say that you will experience life "as it is" with this easy practice. But, deepening your practice into any kind of meditation is a process that requires time and you shouldn't go to a meditation session with a preconceived notion.

It can be practiced from any posture you prefer, whether sitting down or lying down. Make sure you're at ease.

1. Eyes closed. It is possible to use the use of an eye mask to help with this situation, because we would like to see only as much radiation as we can.

2. Relax for a few breaths out and in like I've mentioned previously and take your time letting your muscles ease from head to foot.

3. Be aware, but do not focus upon the darkness or the lack of illumination. The feeling should be comfortable and not frightened or discomforting. Keep in mind that it's the lack of light that permits light to exist, much like the sound needs silence. These are the places which everything is made from and everything that's produced could ever exist without them.

4. Take note, but don't fixate upon the variations that occur in the dark. The object could move, or even swirl around. Simply let

it happen in a state of no reaction. Don't follow the pattern or move. Take note of the movement.

5. There is a chance that you will notice the light or color at a certain point. Again, you can just let the light to pass through while allowing your mind to remain completely empty.

6. If you are able to practice this method, you might be able to experience a brief moment of complete silence thoughts. The reason for this is the silence of the mind, neutrality and absence of any reaction. The longer you are able to observe and then not respond to the "no thought" experience the closer you will be to your root. You are the "you" behind the you.

7. Perform this practice for the length of time or as short as you want, whether that's five minutes, twenty minutes, or even longer.

This is the entire exercise. Enjoy.

Counting

This is among my most favored meditations because of its simple nature. If I'm trying to get my thoughts out of my head and be free of thoughts, it's something that is almost impossible to achieve. Therefore, trying to concentrate on one aspect is the best alternative, except if you're a pro.

One thing I'll concentrate on is taking breath count. Every time I exhale, I'll add 1 to the number between 1 and 10. If I get to 10 I'll begin with 1. This keeps me much more focused rather than keeping track of up and down & simpler numbers are much easier to remember.

If you go over 10 (and most likely are likely to) simply start over at 1 whenever you realize. If you don't remember what the number is simply pick a number, and then keep going.

A routine for your brain to concentrate on can calm the mind. It can be complicated, however you might have a mental overload while you count. As you count it is possible that you do not be aware of it taking place. As always, when this happens, you need to refocus.

Do not be ashamed of being a little agitated. It's a reaction and we're practicing non-reaction and neutrality to the very best of our abilities. Restart counting, and then keep the silence between. Simple, yet effective.

Meditation in multi-phases

A multi-phase mindfulness is a type of meditation which involves paying attention to different subjects or aspects during the various stages of practice. Each stage could have an emphasis or goal like meditation, relaxation, or meditation.

If you spend a couple of minutes on one moment, it helps prepare you for the following phase and create a stronger and effective routine overall.

Here's a four-phase meditative which I have found to be quite helpful.

Phase 1: Relaxation, breathing and clearing the mental clutter (5 minutes)

1. Find an appropriate sitting or lying place. Relax your eyes, and take several deep breaths, focussing on the feel of your breath as it flows between your body. Make sure you breathe deep into the stomach.

While breathing and breathe, you should try to get rid of all thoughts and distractions that are on your mind. Imagine your thoughts as clouds that move through your thoughts, then be able to observe them and not get lost in them.

While continuing breathing, you should try to calm each area of your body. Begin with your feet, and work toward the top of your head.

Phase 2: Gratitude (5 minutes)

Think of the people who did things for you and that you're happy for. Imagine these individuals in your thoughts and take some time feeling thankful of their contributions to your everyday life.

You could also think of specific acts the people you admire did for you and then allow yourself to appreciate and feel grateful for the actions they have taken.

Phase 3: focusing on a goal for the future (5 minutes)

Recall an idea or goal which you'd like to achieve in the coming time. It might be a private target, like improving your fitness or acquiring the latest skill but it may also be that is related to your job or relationship.

When you think about your goal, attempt to believe that you've already accomplished the goal. Keep the feeling of appreciation and gratitude from earlier in the process when you think about. Visualize what it will be as if you had achieved this point, allowing you to feel these emotions.

Remember that it's okay if you aren't able to see the image you're trying to picture inside your mind's eye. The most important thing is your feeling.

Phase 4: Getting insight (5 minutes)

Take some more deep breaths, then bring your attention to the inside. While you breathe, attempt to release your expectations and preconceived notions regarding the kind of insight you could get.

Note any thoughts or emotions you have, then be aware of them, without judgement. It is possible that you will discover new ideas or thoughts appear spontaneously when you remain in this open mind, open state. If it doesn't work to you, it's completely fine. Let the ripples of the meditation to occur when they happen.

I hope this will help! There are apps such as Calm to schedule alarms to each phase of meditation If you'd like.

Open Eye Meditation

Though most of us consider meditation to be a practice that requires the eyes shut There are many people who practice who meditate with their eyes wide open. Based on what I've read meditation with your eyes wide can provide some advantages which closed eyes don't enjoy. If you shut your eyes, you're blocking the senses that you are using and allowing you to have fewer stimuli that you are able to process. It can help you to focus your attention and focus less but, once you return to normal activities, you'll be surrounded by visual stimuli. Even though closing your eyes can help calm you down, it won't necessarily help to practice mindfulness when "life stuff" comes up.

While you are practicing your meditation with eyes closed and your eyes open, you can make the external environment a an integral part of your practice however, in many situations you're restricting the focus of your eyes to a narrow area. This can help you stay focussed on what is happening rather than absorbed in thoughts about the future or past. Additionally, it can assist you to remain aware of the world around you all day long.

By meditatively opening your eyes this can remind you that your everywaking times can serve as even a time of meditation. There is no need to cover your eyes in order to reach that state of calm. It can provide you with tools to ease anxiety and feel at ease in all situations. While there are certain advantages to exploring your own inner self through closed-eye meditation, when you open your eyes and your eyes wide, you can create a deeper relationship between yourself and the external world.

Chapter 5: The Wall Gazing Meditation

Meditation on the wall is an easy but powerful method of focusing your attention to a specific location, which is usually in a wall or another surfaces. This is an effective technique to increase focus, clarity as well as inner peace. How to perform the wall-gazing meditation:

1. You should have a wall, or any other level surface that's at eye-level.

2. The goal is to get closest with the wall is possible. Two feet or less is the ideal distance.

3. Relax your eyes and breathe deeply to ease your mind and calm yourself.

4. Once you're done, close your eyes and look at a wall you've selected. Then, you can look at a small scratch or crack on the wall. Or, you may simply gaze at an empty area.

5. When you are looking at the location, attempt to focus your gaze and unflinching.

Naturally, your mind will begin to wander. If you begin to notice that your thoughts are drifting take a moment to bring your focus to the location.

6. Begin to stare at the location until you are comfortable. Typically, this is five to twenty minutes. Set an alarm or use an app that helps you record your duration.

7. If you're ready to stop your meditation, close your eyes, and breathe deeply. Sit in silence and observe any shifts within your mind or body.

Meditation on the wall can be an effective method for fostering the ability to focus and to find inner peace. Take your time and persevere because it may take some time for you to master the ability to remain focused. After a few sessions, you'll observe that meditation on the wall gets easier and more effective as time passes.

Candle gazing

Meditation with a candle is a method of focussing your attention on only one thing, for example it is the flame from the candle. It is a great technique to increase focus, clarity and inner peace. This is how you can do an enlightening candle meditation:

1. Set a candle on eye level and about 1 meter from your face.

2. Relax your eyes and breathe deeply to calm and relax.

3. If you're all set, open your eyes to look at the burning candle. It is possible to focus your attention on the whole flame, or on a particular part for instance, the tip as well as the base.

4. When you look toward the burning flame you must try to focus your eyes on the flame. Your mind is likely to wander. Similar to all kinds of meditation, it is important to slowly bring your focus back to your goal.

The practice of gazing at candles is believed to boost the pineal gland (also called the third eye) and also to open psychic capabilities.

Meditation during walks

Meditation is a method which focuses on the experience of walking along and the environment around you in order to develop awareness and the state of relaxation. This is how you can practice a walk meditation:

1. Choose a peaceful, quiet area to walk in like the park or the garden. A place that is less crowded

2. Start slowly and walk in a relaxed, natural speed. Be aware of the feeling of every step, the motion of your feet and the touch to the surface.

3. While walking, make sure to remain aware of the surroundings. Be aware of the

sights, sounds and scents as well as the sensation of the sun's air on your skin.

4. If you find your mind wandering to the side, gently draw your attention to the experience of walking, and to your present. It is possible to use an affirmation or simple word, like "left foot, right foot," to keep your focus.

5. You can continue moving and focusing on mindfulness whatever time you'd like. You are able to take a walk for a specific amount duration, or until you are comfortable and at peace.

Walking meditation is an excellent way to develop the state of mind and relax within your everyday life. It's an easy and relaxing exercise that you can do any time, anywhere. This is the only form of meditation that requires movement in the nature. Therefore, it can be an effective method to ease stress in contrast to sitting, which may require greater patience in order to achieve the state of relaxation.

Meditation for the peripheral

Peripheral Vision Meditation is a method of paying attention to the peripheral, or edge of your field of vision. It's a wonderful method to develop meditation and relax. Learn how to perform an eye-to-eye meditation:

1. Choose a comfy sitting place and go through the muscles relaxation.

2. If you're ready, close your eyes and look directly ahead. Let your focus grow to the outer edges of your vision field not focusing on something in particular. If this does not seem natural to you, then hold your index fingers the front of you and gradually pull them apart and focus your attention with your eyes closed. It's just focusing your eyes. After you've completed this procedure, you're able to reduce your arms and continue in the exercise.

3. While you stare with your eyes that are peripheral, make sure to remain aware and present to the world around you. Pay attention to the shapes, colors and movement within the peripheral of your vision field not attempting to concentrate upon any particular object.

4. While practicing peripheral vision It is important to not identify or label any object that you observe, but just let them remain as they are. That means that you let away the desire to label, categorize or make sense of what you see as well as allowing objects to exist within your vision field.

5. If you find your mind wandering at times, slowly bring your focus back to the outer edges of your field of vision.

6. Keep practicing your peripheral vision meditation until you are comfortable. Typically, this is between 5 and 20 minutes. Set an alarm or use an app for meditation to monitor your time.

If you can practice not labeling or making judgments about the things that you observe in your peripheral in meditation, you'll develop an attitude of acceptance and openness to the world around you. This could lead to more concentration and relaxation and a stronger feeling of being in your present.

Mindfulness

Mindfulness and meditation are commonly employed interchangeably but do not mean the exact identical. The practice of meditation is usually sitting at a distance or walking, being aware. It's more about focusing on your normal activities everyday and remaining attentive with the current moment.

Some mindfulness techniques to attempt are:

Mindful eating: This method is about paying focus on the sensations of food that enters the body, and observing the distinct flavours and the textures.

"Mindful Listening": The method requires you to pay attention to sound around you, whether they're music, nature or people speaking. Focus only on the sound, instead of getting caught up in your thoughts on it.

"Mindful movement": The method is about incorporating mindfulness into exercise like yoga, tai-chi or stretching. While you move, attempt to concentrate on the feeling of your body and move itself rather than losing yourself in thoughts.

It is also possible to be aware when washing dishes, doing laundry, or preparing your mattress. Every opportunity to be aware of your actions and not judge yourself is the definition of mindfulness.

Incorporating mindfulness into your routine can enhance relations, improve self-awareness as well as create a better satisfaction and sense of purpose throughout the world. The research has proven that meditation practices help lower blood pressure, boost sleep quality, and lessen the pain that comes with chronic illness. Additionally, it can be beneficial for managing certain conditions, such as anxiety, depression, as well as post-traumatic stress disorder (PTSD).

Another advantage is that it permits people to tackle issues with a focus and clarity. This can lead to more informed choices, which can increase imagination and creativity.

Implementing mindfulness-based practices to your daily routine may be as easy as taking only a few moments each day to pay attention to your breathing or pay focus on the present. It's likely that you'll notice an improvement in your overall well getting better pretty fast.

Holding Space

The act of holding space can be a potent method of meditation that can prove very beneficial for the person who is holding space and the person who is receiving it. It's about creating a comfortable atmosphere that is supportive and in which the emphasis is upon being present and focussing on the other person with no any judgment or interruption. By holding space, you're providing your attention, presence as well as compassion. This will help the person feel loved, supported and validated.

When two individuals engage in the act of occupying space, they have the chance to create a profound connected, mutual connection. When each participant takes turns taking space for their partner in essence, they offer their attention and presence to each other as a gesture of love as a result it makes them more attentive as well as attentive and caring their own. Sharing this experience together can lead to an intense sense of security and security.

If two people participate by taking space, it creates an opportunity for the energy of one can be felt by another in a reverse manner. It also helps to let go of stagnant or obstructed energy, leading to greater feelings of wellbeing and energy. If we are able to hold the space of another in this way, we create an environment for sharing energy exchange.

The advantages of holding space may go beyond doing exercises with a partner. The practice can have ripple effects as every person is more attentive attuned, sensitive and more able to show how they show in their relationships and their daily lives.

Manifestation

Manifestation

It is the process of creating your ideal outcome into realisation through an influence of thought as well as your beliefs and decisions. This involves setting clear goals and imagining the desired result as well as taking the necessary steps to achieve it.

In contrast to cleansing your mind of any thoughts such as meditation does the practice of manifestation, such as visualization, is a goal that you imagine in your mind. It is important to be as precise as you possibly can in creating your plans as well as to ensure you're aligned to your ideals and beliefs.

The process of manifesting involves forming the mental picture of the outcome you want to achieve Imagine yourself in your desired position and concentrate on the thoughts and feelings that are associated with the situation. The more realistic and vivid your visualization is, the better it will be in aiding you in achieving your dream result.

A method to get your mind and heart into believing something which isn't possible in current real world is to focus on the sense of reaching your goal. The process involves taking on the emotion and thoughts of having accomplished their goals.

If, for instance, you want to create an effective business, try experiencing the feelings of pride as well as happiness and achievement like your company has already been profitable. This can help bring your focus to the goal, and helps your goal feel more realistic.

Another option is to concentrate on being grateful for what you have already around you that match with your goals. If, for instance, you want to create an intimate relationship it is possible to practice being gratitude for the affection and bond which you have already throughout your day whether with relatives, friends, or your pets. This can help change your attention from insecurity to a sense of abundance. This will make the goal seem easier to achieve. Be focused on the little wins and the positive change you are experiencing already throughout your day. The same feelings that you'd like to manifest the things you want to achieve.

It is best to avoid focusing on the entire process for achieving your goal rather, concentrate on the end result, or the end goal. The "how" work itself out allows the energy that manifests within the universe the ability to determine the most effective route for you.

Scripting

This is an excellent method of manifestation that is effective in creating goals and dreams in my life. It was developed through Neville Goddard, who is probably the most well-known individual in the field of manifestation. It's a new twist on manifestation which takes some minutes to complete, but it requires a little bit of preparation.

Instead of just thinking about things you'd like to do from out of the air, we're rather going to write the "scene" or a set of events that can only occur if the desired outcome has already been accomplished.

If, for instance, we were looking for a particular car, you could imagine being in the vehicle with a companion and your friend commenting "I love your new car!" And you reply "Me too! I'm almost shocked to discover it's mine!"

This script must be brief, which means it can be remembered and created quickly and without any errors. The "scene" should only take only a few minutes to develop through your mind. Make sure you take your time in creating your ideal short-form scene to achieve the goal you want to achieve, since the process can be challenging to master without planning.

Do not put too much emphasis on the way you'll get your desires. Let the universe figure it out.

Once you've written the scene, you enter in a state of meditative relaxation and repeat the scene repeatedly until it is real to you. You should try to integrate all your senses.

It's the smell of a new car and the sound of conversations being able to feel the steering wheel.

When this sequence becomes repeated enough times to be real to you, take the confidence that you've captivated your subconscious mind. Let it go. You can go about your daily routine without thinking about it. Allow the universe to perform its job as it pleases. If you follow this procedure correctly just once, that's all it is required.

The thought of focusing on your goal is the message to your mind that you aren't sure that it's possible and aren't certain that your goal will come to your own in time.

The Listing Method

It's a basic routine that can make it effortless to integrate the big and small in your day-to-day. It's efficient as it allows you to release and enjoy enjoyment with it.

It's really easy. It's all you require is two things: a notebook and a pen. Making notes by hand is the best way to go because it is stimulating both the mind and body.

Everyday you'd like to record at least 10 things that you'd like to come in your life. Like most manifestation techniques the practice of creating declarations in the present tense like you have something you're looking for.

Do not overthink your decisions and don't be too serious about things. Keep the larger things in perspective by incorporating enjoyable small-scale aspects.

In this case, you could write "I receive a free cup of coffee", "I get a hug from a stranger", "I see a siamese cat" or "I pass someone on the street wearing a cape" in addition to "I love my new 4 bedroom house".

When you are making your list, be yourself consider things you'd like to do. After you're finished and have completed your list, don't look back at the list ever again. Create a new checklist each day and try not to make the same mistakes.

In the next few months there will be 100's, or maybe 1000's of notes that you've written down and mostly neglected. Do not worry about how the events develop or how long it could require. It's not your responsibility. Only your job is to make your list.

As time passes, you'll begin to see things you jotted down come to realization. Be careful not to break the spell trying to justify why some events could be happening even if you didn't record it.

While there are certain circumstances that can appear in seemingly unimaginable ways however, the majority of things manifest in a way that they don't seem like magic at all. Don't question it & don't obsess. Simply make it a pleasant everyday routine, and you might realize that you're much stronger than you imagined.

Chapter 6: What Is Mindfulness Meditation?

The practice of mindfulness meditation is one type of meditation which focuses upon being fully present and present in the moment. This is a method of meditation which allows a person to be conscious of emotions, thoughts, and feelings without judgment or attachment. It helps create a sense of inner harmony and peace.

The practice of mindfulness meditation has its roots in Buddhist philosophical thought and has been practised throughout the ages. It's a means to become aware of the present moment and examine one's feelings and thoughts in a non-judgmental and detached manner. Being aware of your emotions, thoughts, and emotional state, a person is able to gain insight into their personal self-awareness and gain more understanding of themselves and their thoughts and feelings.

Meditation with mindfulness has become more fashionable in recent years, because growing numbers of people taken an interest in its positive effects. Studies have shown that meditation with mindfulness can help decrease stress, increase concentration, and can even boost awareness of oneself. There are a variety of forms of meditation that focus on mindfulness. However, the majority of them involve focusing upon an object or sound that is calming, like the breath as well as letting thoughts flow and disappear without judgment or an attachment.

The advantages of mindfulness meditation are able to be felt physically as well as mentally. Physically, mindfulness practice can lower stress levels, boost the immune system as well as improve sleeping patterns. In terms of mental health, mindfulness meditation may assist in decreasing anxiety, increase concentration and improve self-awareness.

Meditation for mindfulness isn't difficult to master, however it requires time and effort. It is crucial to find an area that is quiet and comfortable for practice that is free of distracting factors. Also, it is essential to be kind and patient as you learn mindfulness meditation. The ability to stay at the present moment requires some time and effort and practice, but it's well worthwhile.

Meditation with mindfulness is an effective instrument that will give you the feeling of inner tranquility and equilibrium. It helps to lower stress, enhance focus and enhance awareness of oneself. Focusing only on the present by observing the thoughts and feelings without judgment or attachment, an individual will gain a better comprehension of themselves as well as a greater connection to their own self.

Benefits of Mindfulness Meditation

Meditation with mindfulness is an effective method of meditation which offers multiple benefits to those who practice it. This practice assists in developing a better awareness of oneself and the environment around them. The practice of mindfulness meditation has been shown to enhance mental and physical well-being, decrease stress levels improve focus and concentration and increase awareness of oneself.

Meditation that is based on mindfulness can help decrease anxiety and stress levels. Research has shown that mindfulness meditation can reduce the stress response of your body which can lead to a sense of calm and improved well-being. It also helps to decrease the frequency and intensity of negative thoughts and allow the mind to concentrate at the present.

The practitioners of mindfulness meditation have reported higher levels of concentration and focus. Focusing on the task at hand can allow people to manage their work and be more efficient. In addition, it helps to increase concentration when faced by a challenging tasks. It is also proven to lower the likelihood of developing disorders such as anxiety and depression.

Meditation with mindfulness can enhance awareness of oneself. It is a great way to draw awareness to emotions and thoughts, which allows people to develop a greater awareness of their own environment. In addition, mindfulness can assist in increasing one's ability to let go of their thoughts and feelings, which allows the person to see them without judgement. It can help in learning to recognize triggers and help the person to control the reactions they experience.

Additionally, meditation with mindfulness may aid in increasing compassion and empathy. This can lead to an understanding and compassionate behavior towards others and oneself. This is particularly beneficial in relationships. It can allow individuals to have a greater comprehension of the feelings and desires.

Through mindfulness it can help one gain better understanding of oneself and the world around them. This can aid in reducing anxiety and stress levels, boost concentration and focus, as well as improve awareness of oneself. In addition, it helps develop compassion and empathy, which allows to build stronger relationships with other people. Therefore mindfulness meditation can be an effective tool that is able to improve your inner peace and well-being.

Preparing to Practice Mindfulness Meditation

Meditation through mindfulness is a path toward inner peace. But prior to beginning this journey, it is essential to be sure the route ahead is easy and secure. This chapter will outline how to get ready for mindfulness meditation.

The initial step is to locate a quiet and comfortable place. It is essential to select the right place to be able to relax and unwind without interruptions. This can be in the bedroom, living space, or even a garden bench. It's a good idea to organize the area by putting in a couple of things including a cushion or chair or blanket, as well as the timer.

The third procedure is to select the time of day that one is able to meditate uninterrupted. It may be beneficial to schedule a specific period of time during the day or each week to engage in mindfulness practice. It will aid in establishing an established schedule.

The final method is to develop the most comfortable position. A straight and upright spine is the best way to practice mindfulness meditation. It is possible to relax on cushions, a cushion, or even the floor. It's important to remain at ease, yet not too as to be so comfortable one could be prone to falling asleep.

Fourth step is to pay attention to breathing. It is possible to do this through taking a breath count or by simply watching the breath. It is important to remain aware of your breath and in order to see it clearly without judgment or distraction.

The final method is to become mindful of any emotions or thoughts that may arise during your process. It is crucial to not be judging yourself and just take note of the thoughts and feelings. If you find yourself getting distracted by emotions or thoughts, just bring themselves back to their breath.

In the end, the final thing to do is to do some practice over the specified period of time. It's useful to start by practicing for only a couple of minutes before moving toward longer-term sessions. The aim is to develop the habit of regular practice and maintain the practice.

If one follows these steps, you can start preparing for a path to tranquility through mindfulness meditation. The chapter in this article has discussed the ways to begin preparing for the practice of mindfulness. In the following chapter, we'll discuss the advantages of mindfulness and ways to integrate mindfulness into your daily routine.

Chapter 7: Breathing Techniques

Breathing is among the main elements that mindfulness meditation has to offer. When practiced regularly you can use it to achieve a state of tranquility and calm. This chapter will explore the various breathing techniques that can be utilized to achieve the state of peace within.

The primary technique is diaphragmatic breathing. It is characterized by breathing deep through the nose, and then out of the mouth. It is important to focus upon the chest and stomach while breathing into and out. This kind of breathing can help to reduce heart rate and ease anxiety.

The other technique is abdominal breathing. The technique involves taking slow deep breaths through the nose and out via the mouth. Concentrate in the abdomen when breathing is carried into and out. This kind of breathing can help to ease tension in the body as well as ease tension.

The third method is known as four-part breathing. The technique is to breathe in deep and slowly through your nostrils, for a period of four. In the next step, you hold your breath for the duration of four. Inhaling slowly from the mouth to count four. Finally, pause to count four. This breathing technique can slow the heartbeat, and induce an overall feeling of peace.

The fourth technique is known as alternate nostril breathing. The technique requires breathing slow and deep through one nostril, and breathing out deeply and slowly through the opposite nostril. Your focus should be on breathing when it is moving through the nostrils. This breathing technique can help to regulate both hemispheres of your brain. It also reduces anxiety and stress.

Fifth technique is known as progressive relaxation. This method involves tensing, and then releasing various muscle groups throughout the body. It starts at the feet before moving towards the face. It is important to focus on the feeling and relaxation that comes from every muscle group. This breathing method assists in relaxing the body and relieve tension.

This is just one of the various breathing techniques that are employed to attain a sense that is peaceful and tranquil. Regularly practicing these breathing techniques will aid in achieving feelings of peace and calm. If you keep practicing this technique will grow simpler and more efficient.

Body Scanning

Body scanning is a vital element the practice of meditation that is mindfulness. It's the act of paying attention to each area of your body with a methodical manner and allowing the body ease and the mind to be calm. It's a method to assist us in becoming aware of our bodily sensations as well as our emotional and mental state.

The body scan starts by focus on breathing to allow the breath to flow naturally and easily. Next, attention shifts to the feet, paying attention to any sensations that occur in the feet. The attention then moves through the body, taking note of any sensations that arise in the hips, legs the chest, abdomen fingers, neck forehead, and the face. As attention is moved up to the upper body part, the person observes any sensations which arise and acknowledges them with no judgement.

After the practitioner is able to move their focus up to the body and then back down, they are able to shift their focus back to the body, and notice any variations in body sensations. This can be done many times. The key is to remain in the present moment and avoid being lost in thoughts or feelings.

The body scan is employed as a method to aid us in becoming conscious of our mental and physical state of mind. This can assist us in be more conscious of our bodies, our moods, and thinking. It also helps us become more aware of our moods and how they impact the physical and mental state of our bodies.

The body scan could also serve to aid people unwind. Focusing on the body, and allowing it to let itself relax, we will be able reduce stress and tension within the body. It can also help us improve our mindfulness, enabling us to remain more at the present moment, and to be more mindful of our emotions and thoughts.

Body scanning is possible at any angle that you are comfortable in including standing, sitting, as well as lying on your back. It is essential to remain relaxed and do not try to force something. It is equally crucial to be soft and not to push your body too much.

When we regularly practice movement, we be more aware and mindful of our bodies, our experiences, as well as our thinking. It is possible to become more tuned to our mental and physical state, which allows us to be relaxed and fully present.

Working With Thoughts

Thoughts are powerful and frequently cause us to behave in specific manners. Meditation helps us be aware of our thoughts, and also be able to observe them without judgement. It lets us be able to step back and look at our thoughts, rather than being in control of them.

In the course of the practice of mindfulness, it's crucial to keep in mind that thoughts aren't actual facts. They're just thoughts that pass through the mind, and are not to be viewed as factual. It is crucial to keep in mind that the thoughts we think about can be affected by our beliefs as well as external influences.

The aim of meditation with mindfulness is to be conscious of our thoughts, and observe their thoughts with no attaching. This isn't an easy thing to master, because it is a process that requires a lot of the practice. It is nevertheless feasible to increase our awareness of our thoughts, by being aware of when and why they come up as well as how they influence our moods and behaviors.

While practicing mindfulness, it's crucial to be patient in our relationship with ourselves, and release judgment. Self-compassion training helps us become gentle and compassionate with the thoughts we have, instead of making judgments about them. It is done by being aware of the thoughts we have without attaching any value to them.

Also, it is important to develop a non-judgmental approach to observation. It is about observing your thoughts and not making them into positive or negative. It allows us to be more conscious of our thoughts and not be affected by the thoughts.

It is important also to develop present-moment awareness. It's done by being aware of the present moment, and then observing the thoughts of our mind without attaching any significance to these thoughts. This will help us increase our awareness and mindfulness of our thoughts and feelings without getting influenced by the thoughts.

It is also essential to learn acceptance and release. It is accomplished through accepting thoughts and feelings without judgement and letting them go with no adhering to them. It can assist us in get more conscious of our thoughts, and look at them with a clear mind.

Through these methods by practicing these techniques, we will become more conscious of our thoughts, and more aware of our feelings as well as our behavior. It can assist us in learning to improve our awareness and attain inner peace.

Chapter 8: Emotions

They can become a dominant factor in our lives influencing how we view and engage with our surroundings. The ability to deal with emotions can be an effective instrument to find inner peace and harmony. The practice of mindfulness meditation is a wonderful method to begin.

The practice of mindfulness meditation helps us be aware of our emotions and not judge them and allows us to observe your feelings and not get too caught up with their emotions. It allows us to take an uninvolved step and see things from a different clarity. You can see your emotions more objectively and with more understanding. It is also possible to be conscious of how our feelings and thoughts influence the other, and the ways in which our behaviour is dependent on them.

Meditation on mindfulness helps us be aware of our emotions and be aware of the triggers behind them. Then, we can choose to be more creative, instead then reacting in the same manner we are. This could help us get out of the negative habits and to create positive patterns of living.

A practice of mindfulness helps us be more accepting of us. You can develop the ability to recognize the emotions we feel without judgment, which allows us to accept your feelings and not be overcome by the emotions. This helps us keep our connection to ourselves as well as to those around us, even in tough moments.

When we engage in mindfulness meditation and mindfulness, we also come to the realization that it's possible to discern when our emotions do not serve our well. Learn how to release harmful emotional attachments as well as to let go of keeping a hold of old wounds. This helps us progress with greater freedom and peace.

Meditation with mindfulness is a powerful method for dealing with emotional issues. It assists us in observing your feelings and thoughts without judgement. It also helps in order to develop a greater compassion for us, and recognize that our emotions are not helping our best interests. Through practice, we will be able to discover our inner peace and harmony.

Working With Sensations

In this section, students are taught how to deal with the body's sensations and develop a sense of inner tranquility. Meditation with mindfulness can lead to an increased awareness of oneself and an in-depth examination of your body's physical feelings. It can serve as a useful tool for creating inner peace and feel more at peace.

The practice of working on sensations begins by being aware of your body. It is accomplished by being aware of physical sensations, such as the sensation of pressure, temperature tension, or additional subtle sensations. While the body is examined, focus is paid to areas that feel particulary tense, painful or discomforting. It is vital to keep in mind that no judgement should be given to these sensations as it is best to look them over with a sense that is open.

In this way you can be aware of the sensations and classify them according to the degree of intensity that is moderate, mild, or even intense. When one is aware of the strength of the feeling then one is able to investigate the feeling and the effects it has. The process involves taking note of the thoughts and feelings generated by the experience and how they affect the body.

Next, you need to take the time to be in touch with the experience. It is possible to do this by simply focusing on the sensation while allowing it be what it is, not striving to alter the experience. It is possible to observe gently the physical changes within the body when the feeling is felt. The process may help lessen the intenseness of the feeling and allows the body to experience a more relaxed sense of calm and acceptance.

In the end, you can try to let go of the sensation. The method involves focussing on breathing and letting the feeling disappear. While breathing in it, tension will be let go and the feeling can be more subtle. As each breath is taken the feeling can be let go to be replaced by the feeling of calm.

The process of working with the sensations is able to be repeated whenever necessary and will help increase the sensation of tranquility and peace. In allowing your body to let go, the mind can get more in touch and conscious of the moment. Through this increased awareness, it is possible to begin exploring the world of one's own and experience a feeling of calmness within.

Working With Images

Images that are visual is a potent instrument for mindfulness meditation. Images offer a vivid visual representation of the inner world. Images can help concentrate on the present as well as to clarify the mind, and aid in achieving a feeling of peace within.

When dealing with images, you must be aware of the images you are creating. It is crucial to pick images that have meaning and are positive. The visualization of positive images may help people to feel feelings of calm. In addition, it helps to be able to pay attention to the picture until it is crystal clear and vibrant.

Another way to utilize images for mindfulness is to fix your attention on a particular object or a scene. The image could come like a natural scene, an artwork or another image that has meaning and is positive. It is possible to spend just a couple of minutes looking at the picture and allow oneself to become absorbed into the image.

This can help bring an inner calmness and peace within.

Another method of working with images is using guided imagery. It is the practice of focusing on an image that has been led by a trainer or a practitioner. It can create a feeling of peace and clarity. In addition, it could assist in bringing an individual's growth and transform.

In addition, imagery could be utilized in a more imaginative way. In particular, you can make use of images to investigate your inner thoughts. These can aid in bringing to a greater knowing and understanding. Furthermore, it may be utilized to study connections between the mind, body, and the spirit.

When working with images as part of the practice of mindfulness, you can attain a feeling of inner calm and clearness. Images can help concentrate on the present and also to help bring about your personal transformation and growth. In addition, they are a great way to discover the inner world of oneself and enhance one's understanding of himself.

Working With Sounds

The power of sound is an effective instrument for focusing as well as meditative states. It is a great tool to aid in focusing the mind, ease your body and experience an inner sense of calm. The use of sound can help one to focus on the moment in which they are and to settle to a peaceful state easier.

Sound for meditation is a long-standing technique. It's a great method of deepening concentration as well as reconnecting with the inner person. Different strategies and sound effects are used to trigger diverse reactions. The most popular type of meditation sound is a mantra or repeating a phrase or word. The mantra can be uttered loudly or in silence, and may be utilized to assist people stay in the present moment and draw their focus back to the present.

Another kind of music which can be utilized to aid in mindfulness includes guided imagery. It involves listening to stories or visualization. It is a great way to relax or imagine various scenarios, as well as connect to their personal emotions. Music can also be a powerful instrument to enter a peaceful state. Music that is relaxing and is steady in its rhythm will aid in relaxing and entering an euphoric state.

Sound therapy could also aid in bringing awareness of physical feelings. Hearing the sounds of the breath one's self could bring awareness to the body and be utilized to aid in relaxation and connect to their inner self. Additional sounds like waves, or wind could be utilized to awaken the mind to the current the moment.

In the process of working with sounds when working with sound, it's important to have a specific goal and be aware of the intention. It is beneficial to make a environment that evokes certain emotions or emotions. This will help in deepening the experience of meditative. Also, you must remain aware of the amount of sound as well as being conscious of any physical sensations that might be triggered.

The use of sound is beneficial in many ways. It helps one let go and relax into a peaceful state faster in addition to helping to increase concentration and create an inner peace. The use of sound can aid in the awareness of their present, and is a potent instrument to connect with your personal self.

Chapter 9: Silence

The ability to be quiet is among the most effective tools to getting to a place of tranquility. If we just take a few minutes to sit and be quiet and still, we can create inner space to become mindful of feelings, thoughts and feelings. It can be an effective method to reconnect to your inner peace and increase the practice of mindfulness.

Meditation with mindfulness can help us get comfortable with quiet. The practice involves paying attention the breath while focusing on the now. When we do this regularly practice, we will begin to pay attention to the thoughts and emotions of others without any judgment. With time, we'll be more comfortable in the silence we have.

The power of silence can open the door to creative thinking. If we can take time to unwind our thoughts and remain still, thoughts will come to us quicker and more efficiently, and we are able to unleash our potential for creativity. If we're quiet it also allows us to be more mindful of the world around us as well as the beauty that surrounds us.

It's crucial to understand that working in silence can be a challenge. It's possible to get lost in our thoughts. In this case is the case, we must remain gentle with our self and cultivate self-compassion. It is then possible to return the habit of remaining still and peaceful.

It is also crucial to realize that sometimes our brain can be a noisy place. It is possible to feel overwhelmed by thoughts and feelings. If this occurs you may find it beneficial to take a few minutes to be aware of our breathing and become aware of our thoughts and emotions. Then, we can use this awareness to make the space inside ourselves, and start to change our perceptions.

The practice of silence can be an effective way to achieve the inner peace. It can help us be more aware, imaginative and conscious of our surroundings. It's important to realize that this can be a challenge but we can employ self-compassion to keep us in the present. After some practice, we'll become comfortable in the silence, and utilize it to attain the peace within ourselves.

Working With Movement

Meditation through mindfulness is a path toward inner peace. the role of movement is crucial on this path. It can aid us in becoming more mindful of our body's physical and what it requires in addition to helping in establishing a greater connection to the peace within us. Movement is a great way to gain a better understanding into our psychological and mental state, as well as to help us work to clear any obstacles that could prevent us from connected to our own inner peacefulness.

As we exercise mindfully it helps us become more aware of the way we move our bodies, and how it affects our feelings and thoughts. You can notice the physical sensations which arise when we move, and observe how they shift as we move. Also, we can notice any physical tensions or blocks which may be in place, and the way they can be relieved through mindful movements.

In focusing on the movements we make, we will be able to recognize physical sensations within our bodies and what they are related to in our emotional and mental states. This awareness can be used to achieve inner harmony and develop an inner calm. With mindful movements can help us focus our attention on the present moment. This allows us to re-connect to our inner peace, and gain a better understanding of our mental and physical state.

Moving mindfully is a broad concept that can be practiced in many different ways. It is possible to practice mindfulness-based walking as well as yoga, tai Chi or other forms of movement that is a good fit for our bodies. What is essential is to remain aware of your movements and pay attention to any physical feelings that occur in our bodies. You can also utilize mindfulness to overcome any mental or physical blocks that could prevent us from being in touch with the peace within us.

While working with movement it is possible to begin with a moment to pay attention to our breathing and become more conscious of our body. It is then possible moving slowly and taking note of our breath and any other sensations we feel from our body while we move. It is also possible to practice mindful stretching exercises to help let go of any physical tension which may be there.

The practice of mindfulness is the perfect way to reconnect to our inner peace, as well as to increase awareness of our psychological and mental conditions.

Movement can assist us in understanding the obstacles that could be hindering us from being in touch with our tranquility. When we pay attention to our movements and breathing, we will be able to recognize physical sensations in the body, and also to develop a sense of balance within. By focusing on our movements, we will be able to travel toward inner peace.

Working With Nature

Connecting with nature is an effective method for mindfulness meditation. In order to increase awareness of nature the practitioner can utilize nature to help them further their meditation journey. Engaging with nature will help establish a greater relationship with the present and is an avenue to deepen mindfulness.

One of the best methods to connect in harmony with nature is to watch it. By taking a moment to take a look at nature helps bring focus to the present.

Concentrating on the sights, scents and sounds of nature helps to create more mindfulness. It is also beneficial to be in nature for a while by sitting in a quiet spot and watching.

Another method of integrating the natural world is by engaging in mindfulness-based walking. Mindful walking is a type of meditation that involves walking in which you pay attention to the feelings that you experience while walking as well as the surrounding within you. Be aware of the movements that your body makes, how the air feels against your skin, as well as the sound of nature could help in gaining more awareness.

Alongside watching and walking mindfully Mindful eating is also a way to help. The practice of mindful eating is taking note of the experience of eating as well as enjoying the flavor and texture of food. Paying attention to the aromas, colors and taste of food may help bring an increased sense of calm.

In the end, being outdoors can help in developing a sense gratitude and admiration. Spending a moment to take in the beauty of nature's environment can give a deeper feeling of happiness to this moment. Giving thanks to nature's beauty will help bring about more peace and satisfaction.

Being in nature is an essential part of any mindful practice. If you take the time to watch, mindfulness walking, mindful eating as well as expressing gratitude those who practice mindfulness can make use of nature to enhance their meditation. Being in touch with nature helps to create more connection to the present moment. It could be an excellent method to develop greater concentration.

Working With Difficulties

Meditation is a method which helps us become aware of emotions, thoughts and physical experiences. It helps us observe your experiences from a perspective of compassion and understanding. It isn't often easy to stay focused. Problems can take the form of distracting thoughts as well as fatigue, disorientation or frustration.

In the event that we encounter challenges in the course of our work, it's crucial to keep in mind that it is common. These challenges can be a part of growing and learning. Don't be too harsh on ourselves, or expect to get too much out of our practices. It's beneficial to maintain the patience and understanding for ourselves as well as to keep in mind that change is often slow.

It's important to figure out ways to keep yourself motivated even in times of difficulty. Regular training can help keep us on track and may bring about positive change. It is beneficial to break off when necessary or adjust the practice according to our energy levels and needs.

It may also be helpful seeking guidance from a knowledgeable educator or tutor. They might be able to provide advice and assistance, as well as help us keep on track and motivated. They could also supply the tools and strategies to assist us in dealing with our challenges.

Sometimes, it can be useful to second look and consider our work from a greater view. It's helpful to look back at our accomplishments as well as to consider what we've gained. This helps us remain focused as well as to improve the practice we are already practicing.

It is crucial to keep in mind that challenges will always be aspect of growing and learning. It is essential to show the patience and understanding for our own and remember that growth is often slow. By focusing on our attitude it is possible to manage our struggles and achieve tranquility within.

Chapter 10: Pain

The pain is a normal aspect of human existence. It may be physical, emotional or even mental. It may range from minor to extreme. The cause of pain can be an illness, injury or a trauma. But it could also be result of emotional stress or distress. Whatever the reason it is, pain can be chronic and impact the quality of our life.

Meditation with mindfulness can assist us to manage the pain in a calm gentle way. If we are aware of our suffering, we will be able to look at it with no judgment, and have an open mind. So it is possible to be able to acknowledge it and deal with it constructively.

In the case of the pain of an injury, it's important that we remain present to the pain. You can be able to relax and feel the pain and be aware of it, without attempting to modify the experience. You can also focus your focus to our body and pay attention to any symptoms or sensations that come up.

You can try mindful breathing techniques to be conscious and also make space for the discomfort. It is also possible to visualize the discomfort as a wave or clouds, which allows the pain to pass throughout us without becoming trapped.

A different way of dealing with the pain is to work on self-compassion. It is important to remind ourselves that suffering is a part of our lives as well as the fact that we're not the only ones experiencing it. Self-care is also a good practice like getting plenty of sleep, eating a balanced diet and participating physically.

In the end, it is possible to engage in a loving-kindness meditation. This means sending us compassionate and loving thoughts, and wish ourselves wellbeing and peace we would like for other people.

The practice of mindfulness meditation is an effective tool to deal through discomfort. Through observing pain with no judgement, and through practicing self-compassion and loving kindness and compassion, we are able to be able to embrace and accept the discomfort. It is also possible to use mindfulness in order to find our inner strength and strength as well as to discover the way to happiness and wellbeing.

Working With Compassion

Compassion is a crucial aspect of mindfulness. It's an incredibly powerful power that allows us adopt a compassionate as well as a compassionate and understanding approach to life and its difficulties. When we're able to build a sense of empathy towards ourselves as well as the people around us, then we're better able to face difficult situations by showing compassion and empathy.

Mindfulness enables us to be aware of our feelings as well as the experiences of others in our lives, as well as gain a better appreciation of how we can contribute to an environment that is more compassionate. It is evident by the way we talk to other people, the manner in which we engage with them and how we conduct our own self.

As we meditate with mindfulness it helps us become more conscious of our thoughts and emotions and gain a deeper awareness of the needs we have. It also helps us become conscious of the needs of others around us and learn how we can best help the needs of others. Additionally, meditation helps us identify and deal with the causes of our own suffering as well as those of other people.

It is possible to practice mindfulness and assist us in developing more empathy for our own feelings and other people. With the practice of mindfulness, we are able to learn to be more mindful and have a more non-judgmental approach towards our own emotional state as well as those of those around us. This will help us increase our feeling of compassion, tolerance and compassion.

Once we're able to be aware of our own pain and the suffering of others we will be able to see ways to help ease the suffering. The more we are aware of the requirements of others and gain empathy and understanding the needs of others. It is also possible to become conscious of our own needs as well as be more understanding of our own needs.

The practice of mindfulness meditation also helps you develop a stronger feeling of being connected with the world around us. As we become more in touch with the world around us it is possible to be more aware of what we do, say as well as thoughts, and the way they impact others. This will help us develop compassion and empathy for the other.

Through cultivating compassion and empathy through mindfulness, we become more adept at responding to challenging circumstances with empathy and compassion. It is possible to become more mindful of the demands of others in our lives, and better prepared to create more compassionate and peaceful world.

Working With Gratitude

It is a potent method to bring happiness and tranquility to one's life. It's the process of taking note and appreciating little blessings life gives our daily lives. It's a way of expressing gratitude and appreciation for all the goodness that is within our lives, no regardless of how small or big.

The practice of gratitude is a crucial component of mindfulness meditation because it assists in cultivating feelings of connection to the world in all its splendor. It also helps develop an attitude of acceptance that is crucial to achieving peaceful and inner peace. When we express gratitude, we are able to see and appreciate that beauty, joy and joy to be present in our lives even through the toughest moments.

If you are practicing the art of gratitude, you need to pay attention to the goodness that is present every day. Be aware and be grateful for the small things that happen in your life, like a stunning sunset, a humorous joke or even a thoughtful gesture by a loved one. If we concentrate on the positives things in life, we will begin feeling more connected to the world around us and also to ourselves.

For those who want to cultivate gratitude, it's important to make time in the day to reflect on every good thing to be thankful for in our lives. It can be accomplished through meditation, journaling or just taking the time to look back at the positives within one's own life. It's also beneficial to consistently practice gratitude through expressing gratitude to another person. You can do this with simply saying thank you with a smile, an encouraging word or even a hug.

It can be a great way to develop an attitude of appreciation as well as remembering all the wonderful things that happen in our lives. It helps us remain more present and mindful to the present, and recognize that beauty, joy and happiness that is present throughout the day. It can be an effective instrument to cultivate the inner peace and feeling content.

When we make time for gratitude, it is possible to begin to appreciate the blessings and beauty of life, even moments of hardship. When we are more conscious of the positive aspects within our lives, we will begin to adopt an attitude of gratitude and happiness. It is an effective tool that can help cultivate inner peace and tranquility.

Working With Forgiveness

The practice of forgiveness is a crucial aspect of practicing mindfulness. This is usually seen as an arduous process, and many individuals have a difficult time letting go of those who hurt them and even their own. With the aid of meditation and mindfulness it's possible to create a sense toward forgiveness and also allow our hearts to be open to the possibility of understanding healing and change.

Meditation with mindfulness can allow to examine the emotions and emotions that pop up to the surface whenever we reflect on our loved ones who injured us or even our own feelings. The practice can provide us with the ability to look at our feelings, thoughts, and emotions without judgment or attachment. The process may be challenging however it could provide a valuable tool on moving towards acceptance.

The first step when working on forgiveness is to determine the root of the pain. Most of the time, we're focused on the wrong situation or person rather than focusing on the root of the discomfort. If we are able to identify what is causing the pain, then we can start to tackle releasing the pain.

It is also possible to practice mindfulness meditation in order to build empathy and compassion. It can assist us in learning to look at the issue from a different perspective as well as gain insight on our personal experience as well as other people's experiences. Through practicing compassion, we are able to shift away from frustration or anger and develop a mindset that is tolerant and compassionate.

The next step to work towards forgiveness is with self-forgiveness. It can be a challenging method, because it is a process that requires the ability to examine ourselves and admit our mistakes as well as shortcomings. This is however the first step to accepting self-awareness and giving our heart to other people.

In the end, it is possible to use mindfulness to work on acceptance of other people. It can be a challenging method, because it is a process of letting the feelings of anger and bitterness and be able to accept and understand. It is useful to look at the positive aspects of the person and remember that all of us make mistakes, and it's possible to accept forgiveness and make amends.

Through the practice of forgiveness the practice of mindfulness meditation, we begin healing and allow our hearts to open up to possibilities of change. By doing this allows us to love ourselves as well as the other, and create a space for understanding and love.

Chapter 11: Loving-Kindness

Meditation on mindfulness is an effective instrument for cultivating lovingkindness. If practiced consistently the practice can assist people to develop a sense of kindness and empathy towards oneself as well as others. The practice of loving kindness is a crucial part of mindfulness that is a great way to develop an inner peace.

Being a loving person begins by acknowledging that we're all connected, and that we share an innate human being. As we cultivate loving-kindness you develop a awareness of our respect and gratitude to all living things. It also helps us accept and take care of ourselves as well as other people with a non-judgmental attitude.

A practice of loving-kindness is making positive wishes for ourselves and other people. This intention is usually expressed through affirmations or mantras, for example "May I be safe and free from harm" or "May all beings be free from suffering."

The phrases are frequently repeated in meditation, and are used in order to build an attitude of love and empathy.

If you want to be a loving person It is essential to begin with yourself. It is essential to learn to treat our own self with respect and compassion before we are able to extend this kindness towards others. The practice of loving-kindness in order to develop an appreciation for ourselves and self-compassion.

The concept of loving-kindness is also applicable towards those who are around us. The practice of kindness to build an attitude of acceptance and empathy towards other people. It is also a good idea to convey positive thoughts towards those experiencing difficulties or suffering in some manner. Through this method we are able to ease some of their burdens and give them the feeling of security and comfort.

In the end, we can employ the act of kindness to build a sense connection with others. As we cultivate loving-kindness it becomes apparent that we have common humanity as well as the interconnectedness between all living things. Then we realize that we all are members of one world community, and that we have a connection to each other in a certain way.

Through practicing kindness, we will develop a feeling of inner peace, and a sense of connection to the rest of the world. If we are able to embrace this philosophy of kindness, we begin to realize our worth and importance in addition to the importance and value of all living things.

Working With Fear

The emotion of fear is one every person experiences throughout their life. It manifests various forms, from physical sensations as well as mental state. Although fear is an instinctive response to risk or challenging circumstances but it also can be an obstacle to development and growth. Meditation can be an effective tool to deal on fear, and turning it into a positive energy.

Meditation with mindfulness allows us to examine our fear with no judgement or attachement. It is possible to observe the way fear affects the body and observe the way it manifests before passing disappears. Once we have the ability to notice the fear and not engage in the process, we will be able to comprehend it better. It is then possible to employ mindfulness in order to identify what is the root cause of our anxiety and understand our responses to it.

One of the advantages of meditation with mindfulness is that it assists to become more conscious of our thoughts, emotions as well as our emotions. It helps us better comprehend our fears and be aware of when it manifests within our daily lives. Once we have this knowledge it is possible to change our behaviour and attitude in order to manage our fears better.

Meditation with mindfulness can help us develop empathy and compassion towards ourselves whenever we feel fears. This will help us develop more compassion and understanding about ourselves and how we react to fear with a positive way.

When we meditate with mindfulness it can be used to it to develop confidence and courage. It can assist us in learning to confront our fears and then take action in spite of the fear. Mindfulness can help us acknowledge our fears and then decide on the best way to deal with it.

The final point is that mindfulness meditation is a great way to help develop an awareness of inner peace and calm. The practice can help us gain a the feeling of peace and peace, which could assist us in overcoming anxiety and move beyond the fear.

With mindfulness meditation it is possible how to deal with fears with more positive and healthy manner. It can help us increase our knowledge of what we fear as well as to build confidence and courage to conquer the fear. With mindfulness meditation is a way how to control our fears and live an enjoyable and peaceful lifestyle.

Working With Self-Acceptance

Self-acceptance is one that can be powerful. It's a crucial element in the journey to real inner peace. Self-acceptance refers to being able to accept and accepting the self that we have with all its flaws, imperfections and all. It's a way which embraces the whole of yourself, which includes the positive, the negative and the unattractive.

Self-acceptance starts by being aware of your thoughts and emotions. This involves recognizing and paying attention to the thoughts and emotions you experience with no judgment or a sense of attachment. In this way you will begin to understand yourself, and begin to be comfortable with yourself the way you are.

When you are conscious of the thoughts and emotions you experience and thoughts, you will begin to identify certain patterns of your behavior. This will help you find areas in which you might hold onto negative thoughts regarding your self. By doing this you will be able to question these assumptions and substitute them for positive ones.

Self-acceptance can also mean the ability to be a lover of yourself. It means accepting the imperfections you have and learning how to be nice towards self-love. This could mean having breaks as needed as well as setting goals that are realistic and being patient with yourself whenever you do make mistakes. Additionally, you should be nice towards yourself when experiencing negative feelings.

It is crucial to keep in mind self-acceptance is a journey which takes effort and time. It's a long-term process which requires perseverance and commitment. It is crucial to realize that you're not on your own during this process. There is assistance from family, friends or even professionals, if you need it.

Self-acceptance can also be a continual process. It requires constantly challenging your negative thinking and belief in order to replace those with positive thoughts and beliefs. Also, it is vital to be self-care conscious by treating yourself respect and love.

Self-acceptance can be a process which can lead to inner peace. It will help to develop a greater self-awareness and result in a higher confidence in oneself. This can lead to enhanced relationships with people around you as well as better mental health overall. It's a path which can be filled with joy and tranquility.

Working With the Present Moment

Meditation on mindfulness is about living in the moment, accepting whatever happens at any given moment, and then let go of things that does not serve us anymore. In this section we'll look at the significance of working in the present moment, and learn how to effectively do it.

Mindfulness meditation is about becoming conscious of what is happening in the moment with no judgment. This practice can help us achieve greater clarity, focus and a greater understanding of what we experience as well as to make more conscious decisions throughout our lives. This practice allows us to stay aware of our feelings and manage the emotions with skill.

The present moment can be described as an opening to the inner imagination and wisdom. When we are aware of the moment in which we are and allowing ourselves to be open to possibilities available in each and every day. It is possible to choose to put our focus on what is significant and important, and then be embrace the wonder and delight that surround us.

If we are mindful of the present it is possible to let the things that does not serve us anymore. Let off thoughts and beliefs which have held us back, while opening us to the possibility of new possibilities. It is possible to move forward with an awareness of purpose and direction.

The practice of mindfulness meditation can also help develop a sense gratitude to the moment. It helps us appreciate and recognize every moment of happiness as well as beauty and love are experienced. It is also possible to acknowledge and embrace the challenging occasions with understanding and kindness.

When we meditate with mindfulness it helps us to be gentle and understanding toward ourselves as well as individuals and situations that happen within the present. It is possible to practice responding to situations to situations with compassion and love instead of reacting with stress, anger or fear.

The practice of mindfulness meditation can help us make a place of quiet throughout our lives. This space can be used to examine our soul and connect to the essence of who we are. It is a great place to reconnect with our real goal and live in an increased sense of awareness.

In focusing on the now, we can create a feeling of inner tranquility. It is possible to learn to be content with the present moment, give up the things that are no longer serving us, and open to the beautiful and joy at every turn. It is the art of mindfulness meditation.

Working With Goals

The process of setting and reaching goals is an essential part of mindfulness meditation. It's important to set clearly defined, achievable goals order to remain engaged and focused. They can range including simple tasks that are routine to more complex, long-term plans. It's important to be real and break down large goals into manageable, smaller objectives.

In creating goals, it's crucial to keep in mind your goals, and make sure that goals are in line with your values. It's also essential to remain realistic, and not be able to establish targets that are excessively lofty or impossible to reach. After the objectives have been established, it's important to spend time trying to imagine the desired outcome and then create a strategy to achieve the goal.

A practice of mindfulness is extremely beneficial in attaining goals since it aids in gaining concentration, clarity and focus. It can also serve to create an optimistic mental state that can provide the drive and determination needed to achieve one's objectives. Meditation can also help to ease anxiety and stress that can cause anxiety in achieving objectives.

In the process of achieving targets, it's essential to monitor the progress made. It is helpful by breaking goals down into smaller, less daunting assignments and then to mark off each step as it is accomplished. This will help create feelings of satisfaction and is a powerful motivational tool. It is also crucial to remain patient and practice self-compassion. There is a normal feeling of being exhausted and frustrated when striving to reach your goals. But it's important to take time for self-care and recognize every step of your progress.

It is also crucial to keep in mind that goals should be able to change. It is essential to remain flexible and willing to modify goals as required. It is equally crucial to acknowledge the moment when goals are achieved and celebrate achievements. The achievement of goals is an excellent source of satisfaction as well as a powerful opportunity to remind yourself of the benefits of meditation.

Working With Daily Life

The practice of mindfulness meditation can be a potent technique live a life that is more consciousness and presence. This chapter will help you through the process of integrating mindfulness into your daily life. This chapter will teach you how to use your daily routine to create opportunities to develop your own personal development and change.

First, discover how you're responding to your daily life. What is your typical behavior? Are you always rushing through tasks or do you prefer to take time? Do you get easily distracted or do you concentrate solely on the work at hand? Are you critical of you and other people, or allow you and your colleagues the space to be prone to errors?

When you are aware of your tendencies, you are able to begin to address these tendencies. You can do this by reflection on yourself, journaling or mindfulness. Self-reflection is a great way to discover your own habits and patterns. Journaling lets you explore the thoughts and emotions of your mind and is a wonderful instrument for exploring yourself and transforming. It can also assist you to create an environment of openness and acceptance, so you're able to react to your surroundings in a more mindful and conscious way.

The next stage is to discover how to live in the world around us. It is about learning to take in and be present with everything that is going on in the present moment without judgement. It can be a challenge particularly when events don't go as you planned However, with time this will get easier. When you are more in touch in your life, you'll be able to look at the world in a fresh way.

The next step is to develop an mindset of appreciation and gratitude. That means you should take some time to look at the positive aspects of life and take time to be grateful for all the good things, both big and little. It can keep you attuned to the wonder and beauty of life even in difficult circumstances.

Fourth step is practicing self-care. It means that you take proper care of your body the mind, and your spirit. It includes sleeping enough and eating a balanced diet, working out as well as engaging with activities that give you satisfaction.

Fifth stage is to develop an attitude of love and empathy. It is about being considerate and compassionate towards others. It's about being patient and compassionate even if things don't happen as you intended.

It can aid in developing a the feeling of peace within and connections.

When you incorporate these five actions in your everyday life and routine, you will be able to live your life with a mindful and conscious manner. This will allow you to be more conscious and attentive as well as open you up to the possibilities of a whole new world.

Chapter 12: The Benefits That Come From Mindfulness And Meditation

Meditation is proven to offer numerous physical mental and emotional advantages Take a close examine some methods these techniques can enhance the overall health of our lives.

1. Reducing Stress and Anxiety

One of the most widely known benefits of meditation and mindfulness is the ability they provide to lower anxiety and stress. Through mindfulness practices and meditation, we are able to be in the present moment, and get rid of thoughts concerning the future or past. It can allow us to be more relaxed and calm when we are in the middle of difficult situations.

2. Improving Mental Health

Studies have shown that meditation and mindfulness may prove to be highly effective in treating depression and anxiety.

When we learn to be aware of our emotions and thoughts in a non-judgmental manner, we improve our emotional resilience as well as coping abilities.

3. Boosting Immune System Function

Research has also shown that mindfulness practices as well as meditation could increase the effectiveness of your immune system. It could be because of being stressed can weaken the immune system. Also, through reducing stress levels meditation and mindfulness can assist in maintaining the health of your immune system.

4. Enhancing Focus and Concentration

The practice of meditation has been proven to enhance concentration and focus. Through training our minds to concentrate on one area, like breathing, we are able to improve our concentration and mental clarity on our everyday life.

5. Improving Sleep Quality

The practice of mindfulness and meditation can aid in improving sleeping quality. Through reducing stress and encouraging calm, these techniques will help promote the restful and rejuvenating sleep that you need.

6. Increasing Emotional Well-being

Additionally, mindfulness and meditation aid in enhancing general emotional wellbeing. In cultivating a higher level of contentment and peace and a sense of contentment, we will experience more contentment and happiness throughout our lives.

In the following sections, we'll explore the various methods and exercises available to aid you in developing your meditation and mindfulness practices as well as experience the benefits you.

Chapter 13: Understanding The Mind-Body Connection

The body and the mind do not exist as separate entities instead, they're two elements of one. Actually, they're very closely linked that health issues of one is a major influence on the overall health of the one. We'll take a deeper study of the relationship between body and mind as well as how meditation and mindfulness aid in promoting better health and wellness within both of these areas.

1. The Brain-Body Connection

The body and brain are inextricably linked through our nervous system. The brain connects to the body via electrical signals, which flow across the body's nervous system and the body is able to communicate to the brain via feedback mechanisms such as pain and sensation. That means our feelings, thoughts and experiences have an immediate influence on the performance of our bodies, and the reverse is true.

2. The Effects of Stress on the Mind-Body Connection

Stress is among the most significant disruptors to the connection between mind and body. If we are stressed it triggers the body's stress response. can be activated and releases an array of hormones and chemicals that affect everything from our moods to our immune system. In time, prolonged stress may result in a myriad of mental and physical issues.

3. Mindfulness and Meditation as Tools for Health and Well-being

Meditation and mindfulness can assist bring balance back in the body-mind connection through decreasing stress levels and encouraging peace. When we pay attention to the present and fostering a sense of mindfulness and acceptance it is possible to begin shifting our perspective on stress, and enjoy greater health and wellbeing.

4. Techniques for Cultivating Mind-Body Connection

There are a variety of ways to increase awareness of the body-mind connection. One that is most efficient is to use body scanning. In this technique, the focus is on each body part at a time, and then pay attention to the sensations and areas where tension is present. It can assist us in better understand how our emotions and thoughts affect our physical and emotional sensations.

Another technique is mindful breathing, which is when you focus on your breath in order to keep our focus to the present, as well as progressive muscle relaxation which involves systematically tightening and relax every muscle group throughout the body, allowing it to relax tension and encourage relaxation.

If we practice these practices regularly to improve our awareness of the connection between mind and body and feel better overall well-being and health.

How to Practice Mindfulness Meditation

Meditation with mindfulness is an effective method of fostering increased awareness and decreasing stress. Below is a step-bystep guide for beginning mindfulness meditation.

1. Locate a calm and cozy place

Find a place in which you are able to sit comfortably with no distracting factors. It is possible to add chairs or cushions for support.

2. Create an alarm

Create a timer to your preferred duration of exercise. For beginners, it is recommended to begin by practicing for a short amount of time then gradually increase to longer sessions.

3. Begin by deepening your breathing.

Relax for a while to calm the body, and then bring your attention back to your now.

4. Keep your eyes on your breath

Concentrate on the breath sensation when it flows through your body. Some people find it beneficial to concentrate on a specific part of your body, for example the nostrils of your stomach or even your nose.

5. Be aware of the times when your mind wanders.

While you concentrate on your breathing Your mind can be distracted by other thoughts or feelings. It's normal and is natural. If you find that your mind has been wandering, slowly bring the focus back to the breath.

6. Cultivate non-judgmental awareness

When you engage in mindfulness, you should develop a non-judgmental understanding of your thoughts and feelings. Instead of seeking to ward them off or put them down, look at your thoughts and emotions with interest and empathy.

7. Begin with gratitude

As your timer starts to go off, take a couple of deep breaths before bringing the focus back towards your body. You can take a moment to think about the things you're thankful for throughout your day.

8. Make sure to practice regularly

Like all other skills it takes time to master mindfulness. Make it a point to practice each morning, even if it's only for a short amount of time.

Keep in mind that the purpose for mindfulness meditation isn't to completely eliminate emotional or mental thoughts however, rather it's to build an awareness of the experience we have inside us. Through regular practice it is possible to experience greater tranquility, peace and a sense of well-being.

Chapter 14: How To Practice Loving-Kindness Meditation

Love-kindness meditation, sometimes referred to as Metta meditation is a method of creating feelings of compassion, love and empathy towards yourself and other people. How to begin by practicing loving-kindness meditation

1. Locate a calm and cozy place

Find a place that is quiet and free of interruptions. There is a possibility of using an ottoman or a chair to help support your posture.

2. Create the timer

Create a timer to your time frame. For beginners, it is recommended to begin by practicing for a short amount of time then gradually increase to longer durations.

3. Begin by deepening your breathing.

Inhale deeply to relax into the body, and then bring your focus to your now.

4. Make time for someone you love

Think of someone who that you truly love like your family member, companion or your pet. See them through your head, and then begin cultivating feelings of affection and love towards them.

5. Spread love to all

Then, broaden your focus to include other people who are in your lives, like friends, colleagues, or those you might have issues in dealing. Repetition in a quiet way phrases like "May you be happy, may you be healthy, may you be safe, may you live with ease."

6. Develop a love-filled relationship with oneself

In the end, you must bring your focus towards yourself, and then silently say the same words, turning them toward yourself.

This may be difficult for certain people, however it's crucial to engage self-care and compassion.

7. Thank you for your gratitude.

If your alarm goes off, take a couple of deep breaths before bringing your focus towards your body. You can take a moment to think about the things you're thankful for throughout your day.

8. Make sure to practice regularly

Like all other skills, loving kindness is a skill that requires practice. Try to do it every day even if only for a couple of minutes.

The goal of meditation on loving-kindness isn't to instigate feelings of kindness or love instead of cultivating these feelings naturally as time passes. Through regular practice it is possible to experience more empathy, connections and happiness within your daily life.

How to Practice Body Scan Meditation

The body scan meditation is a technique that focuses attention to the various areas of your body and focusing on them in a structured manner. This is how you can practice the body scan:

1. Choose a peaceful and relaxing place

Find a place that allows you to lay on your back or sit in a comfortable position with no distracting factors. There is a possibility of using the cushion or blanket folded to help support your head as well as knees.

2. Create an alarm

Make a schedule for the time frame. For beginners, it is recommended to begin only with a couple of minutes before gradually progressing to longer durations.

3. Start with a deep breath.

Relax for a while to calm your body. Bring your focus to your current moment.

4. Begin by putting your feet on the floor.

Pay attention to your feet, and observe any sensations that you experience, for example sensations of warmth, tingling or tension. Instead of analyzing or thinking about these feelings, just notice these sensations.

5. The body should be moved up

Move your attention slowly to your upper body and bring attention to each body part at a time - abdomen, legs, hips and shoulders, the chest, hands, arms and the head. While you pay attention to every part of your body, note any sensations, tension or movements you feel.

6. Be aware of your surroundings without judgement

When you go through each area that you are in, notice any thoughts or sensations which arise. However, try not to analyze or judge these thoughts. Instead, just acknowledge these sensations and let them pass by directing your attention to your breathing and to the present moment.

7. Begin with a prayer of gratitude

As your timer starts to go off, take a couple of deep breaths before bringing the focus back towards your body. Pause for a few moments to think about the things you're thankful for within your own life.

8. Make sure to practice regularly

As with all skills practice, body scan meditation requires the practice. Try to do it every day even if only for a short time.

A body scan meditation is fantastic way to be aware to your body, and develop awareness and mindfulness. It helps lower anxiety and stress levels and improve your sleep and improve overall wellbeing.

Chapter 15: How To Practice Walking Meditation

Meditation is a method of practice which involves paying attention in the present when walking. Learn how to walk in meditation:

1. Locate a calm and cozy area

Choose a location that you are able to walk around without distracting factors. This could be indoors or outdoors, however be sure to choose a quiet and quiet area.

2. Relax and let your body

Sit still for a few seconds and notice your feet on the ground, the mass of your body and the rhythm of your breathing. Inhale deeply and pay attention to your goal to do a walking meditation.

3. Begin walking gradually

Begin walking at a slow pace, making small steps and paying focus to the sensations of your legs and feet. Notice the motion of your feet when they raise up, then move to the side, only to return to the ground.

4. Be aware of the sensations you feel inside your body

When walking, draw your focus to the sensations that are present in your body. The movement in your legs, shift of your body weight, and the swinging of your arms. Be aware of the thoughts and distracting thoughts that pop up however, try to not get involved with them. Be aware of them and let them go.

5. Use a mantra or visualization

It is possible to employ the power of a mantra or visualisation to focus your thoughts. You could, for instance, say the word "peace" with each step or imagine a serene environment such as the nature or beach.

6. Pay attention to your surroundings

When walking, remain aware of the surroundings. Pay attention to the patterns, colors and patterns of things around you. Pay attention to the sounds of your surroundings or the nature around you.

7. Begin with a prayer of gratitude

Once you're done with the walking exercise, you should take a moment to sit still and observe your body. Inhale deeply and think about the things you're thankful for throughout your day.

8. Make sure to practice regularly

Meditation on walking can be performed in any location and anytime So, try to integrate it into your routine. Just a couple of minutes of meditation will help you develop the habit of mindfulness and ease anxiety.

Walking meditation can be a wonderful option to integrate awareness into your day-to-day activities and to connect to the present. It will help you enhance your mood, boost the awareness you have of the world around you as well as lessen anxiety and stress.

How to Practice Mindful Breathing

It is a straightforward but powerful technique that requires being aware of the feeling of breathing out and in. These are the steps you can follow to take in practicing conscious breathing.

1. Locate a calm and cozy place

Choose a location in which you are able to sit comfortably and not be distracted. This could be a seat mat, cushion or mat. You must ensure that you're at a level and that your spine is straight.

2. Concentrate on breathing

Reduce or close your eyes. your eyes, then bring the focus of your breathing. Pay attention to the sensation of breath moving through as well as out of nostrils or the rising and falling of your stomach or chest.

3. Take note of your thoughts.

While you concentrate upon your breathing You may feel thoughts, emotions, or physical sensations come up. That's normal. Take a moment to notice them and then gently return your focus to the breath.

4. Take a deep breath and count your breaths

For help in focusing your thoughts To help focus your mind, it is possible to take a count of your breaths. Breathe in and slowly begin to count "one," then exhale and count "two." Keep counting until you reach ten and then begin again with one.

5. Take a moment to breathe in.

If you're at ease with counting you may try lengthening your breath. Begin by inhaling for a count of four and exhale after the count of six. Slowly increase the count until you're at ease.

6. Make sure to practice regularly

The practice of mindful breathing is possible whenever and wherever and you should try to do the practice regularly. Begin with only a couple of minutes per day and gradually increment the amount of time until you are at ease.

Meditation can ease anxiety and stress, enhance concentration and focus. It can also help to promote calm and relaxation. It's a straightforward but effective method that you can incorporate in your everyday life that helps you reconnect to your present-day experience and develop the habit of mindfulness.

How to Practice Mindful Eating

The practice of mindful eating which involves paying attention and focus to the sensation of eating. Here are some steps to follow in practicing mindful eating:

1. Set up a healthy eating space

Find a peaceful and relaxing place to sit and eat free of distractions, such as television or a mobile phone. The table should be set with dishes, food items and other equipment you'll require.

2. Enjoy a moment of appreciation for the food you eat.

Before eating, you should take time to take note of the design and smell of the food. Pay attention to the textures, colors and scents.

3. Get your attention on the sensations

Once you're eating take a moment to take your time and engage your senses. In small portions, take your time chewing, paying attention to the tastes, textures as well as the sensations you experience inside your mouth.

4. Keep your eyes on the present

When you are eating, make an effort to pay attention to your present situation. Do not be distracted by thoughts about the past or thinking about the future.

5. Be aware of your appetite and the fullness you feel.

Take note of your body's signals of fullness and hunger. You should eat until you are content, but don't feel too satisfied.

6. Practice gratitude

When you're done your meal, take the time to thank God to your meal and those who helped grow or prepared it, served it, and then enjoyed it.

The practice of mindful eating can help you improve your relation to food, and also encourage mindfulness in all aspects of your life. It also helps aid digestion and decrease eating too much. Through mindful eating you will develop a stronger satisfaction and pleasure when you eat.

Chapter 16: How To Practice Mindful Movement

It is a method of movement that requires bringing awareness and focus on the body's physical sensations as well as movements the body. Below are steps to follow in a mindful practice:

1. Select a practice for movement

Find a workout you like, such as the yoga class, Tai Chi or even walking. You must choose an exercise that is secure and comfortable on your own body.

2. Start by focusing on your breath.

Prior to moving to begin, take some slow breaths. Focus on the sensations of the breath moving through as well as out. It can assist you in learning to be more in the moment and stay centered.

3. Be sure to move with purpose

Once you've started your exercise, do it with intent and concentrate on the physical sensations you experience in your body. Be aware of the muscles you're using and how you breathe, the rhythm in your breathing as well as any places of tension or discomfort.

4. Be present

While moving, you should try to be present and focus upon the sensations that are present in your body. Beware of getting distracted by your thoughts or distracted by distractions.

5. Develop self-compassion

Take care and be gentle with yourself while you are moving. Do not judge yourself for any challenges or limitations which may arise.

6. Then, relax and unwind.

After you have completed your workout for a while, you can take some time to take a break and lie down in a comfy position. Concentrate on your breathing and physical sensations within your body.

Moving mindfully helps you to develop an increased sense of the body's awareness, ease anxiety and stress, and enhance your overall health. Through mindful exercise it is possible to bring greater awareness and mindfulness into the daily routine.

Dealing With obstacles within Meditation Training

Although meditation is beneficial in reducing anxiety and improving your overall well-being, it can be difficult to keep a regular routine. There are a few common challenges which can occur during the practice of meditation and methods for getting over them

1. Boredness or boredom

If you feel unfocused or bored in meditation You can try focusing the focus of your breathing or the area of concentration. Try switching around your practice of meditation through experimenting with new techniques or even incorporating some movements.

2. Physical pain

It's normal to experience uncomfortable physical sensations during meditation like back pain, or a numbness in your legs. If you experience this, consider altering your posture or taking a interval to stretch. Try incorporating the movement into your routine or practice mindfulness of the pain itself.

3. Thoughts wandering

Thoughts that wander are an incredibly common issue in meditation. If you feel distracted, just be aware of the thought, without judgement and slowly bring your focus back to your breathing or to your preferred focus for meditation.

4. Doubt, self-doubt, or criticism

If you're experiencing self-doubt or self-reflection when you meditate, consider doing self-compassion. Accept that those thoughts are common and normal, and then take care to treat yourself with compassion and respect.

5. Inconsistent practice

If you're struggling to maintain an ongoing meditation routine Try setting the time of your morning to meditate. It is also possible to practice in a group, or find an accountability partner who can help ensure you stay on track.

Keep in mind that meditation is a method of practice and you're likely to run into obstacles along the path. When you tackle these hurdles by focusing on curiosity, patience and self-compassion you'll be able to develop a consistent and enjoyable meditation routine.

Developing Compassion as well as Self-Compassion Compassion is the capacity to be aware of and respond to the pain of other people through compassion, empathy and empathy. Self-compassion, on one on the other hand, is the ability to treat yourself with the same compassion as empathy, compassion, and understanding the way one would treat someone who is in a need. Self-compassion as well as compassion are powerful ways of increasing well-being and creating healthy relationships with other people.

Here are a few strategies to developing self-compassion and compassion:

1. Engage in mindfulness with loving kindness

The practice of loving-kindness meditation can be a potent method of cultivating compassion for yourself and other people. When you practice this the focus is on sending good wishes and positive thoughts toward yourself, your loved ones friends, colleagues, or even the people who have possibly caused the harm you suffered.

2. Perform acts of kindness

Simple acts of kindness could help in creating a sense of compassion and understanding for other people. The act of kindness can be as simple as extending a smile to a stranger, or taking time to talk to someone who is in need.

3. Practice gratitude

The power of gratitude is another tool to cultivate self-compassion and compassion. Make time every day to consider your gratitude for the things that you're grateful for and think about expressing gratitude to others too.

4. Practice self-care

Self-care is a crucial element of developing self-compassion. This could mean making time to yourself every day, participating with activities that give you satisfaction and taking care of yourself with compassion and respect.

5. Refrain from the negative self-talk

Negative self-talk is an obstacle towards self-love. If you're caught engaging with self-criticism, or self-doubt Try challenging your thoughts and ask yourself whether they're true or beneficial.

Keep in mind that developing self-compassion and compassion is an ongoing process, which requires time and energy to cultivate. When you incorporate these practices in your everyday life and practice, you will develop an increased sense of compassion and self-compassion and enhance your general well-being.

Chapter 17: Mindfulness And Meditation For Anxiety And Depression

Depression and anxiety are among the most commonly reported mental health issues that impact millions of people across the globe. There are a variety of treatments available the mindfulness practice and meditation may be beneficial tools to manage issues and improving wellbeing.

There are a few ways mindfulness and meditation may help in the battle against depression and anxiety:

1. Develop awareness of thoughts and emotions

The practice of mindfulness meditation can aid people gain a greater awareness of their feelings and thoughts which allows them to identify certain patterns and triggers which could be a cause of depression or anxiety.

2. Have a non-judgmental approach to thoughts and emotions

The practice of mindfulness meditation may also assist people to develop a positive attitude to their feelings and thoughts which can help reduce the effects of self-criticism, negative self-talk, and negative self-talk.

3. Practice relaxation techniques

The practice of mindfulness and meditation can assist individuals to practice methods of relaxation, like deep breathing, and progressive muscular relaxation. This can help reduce the symptoms of anxiety and depression.

4. Improve emotion regulation

The practice of meditation and mindfulness will help people improve their abilities to regulate emotions. This allows people to manage their emotions better and lessen the negative impact of negative feelings.

5. Increase overall wellbeing

Meditation and mindfulness practices will also boost overall health as well as reduce stress and improve the quality of sleep, which could aid in reducing symptoms of depression and anxiety.

It is important to remember that practices of mindfulness and meditation are not a substitute for professional treatments for depression and anxiety. Incorporating these methods as part of a complete treatment plan could be a beneficial approach to control the symptoms and boost overall wellbeing.

If you're suffering from symptoms of depression or anxiety, you should seek out professional assistance with a mental health professional. Along with the practice of mindfulness and meditation You can create an extensive plan for managing the symptoms and improving general well-being.

Mindfulness and Meditation for Better Sleep

Sleeping well is vital to our general health and wellbeing however, many suffer in falling or remaining awake. Meditation and mindfulness practices are effective ways of bettering the quality of and quantity of sleep.

These are a few methods that meditation and mindfulness can aid in achieving better sleep.

1. Lower stress and anxiety

Stress and anxiety create difficulties in falling into sleep and to stay in bed. The practice of meditation and mindfulness are a great way to lower anxiety and stress. They can also help promote more relaxation and a better night's sleep.

2. Improve your relaxation and peace

The practice of mindfulness and meditation will help people develop an inner peace and tranquility, enabling individuals to drift to a restful sleep effortlessly.

3. Create better sleeping routines

Meditation and mindfulness practices are a great way to help you develop better sleeping habits, for example creating a predictable bedtime as well as setting a peaceful bedtime routine.

4. Increase overall wellbeing

The practice of meditation and mindfulness can help improve your overall wellbeing, decreasing stress and improving mood and can lead to a better quality sleep and more of it.

Here are some meditation and mindfulness techniques that are beneficial to improve sleep quality:

1. The Body Scan meditation method involves focusing on the entire body from head to toe and focusing on every part of the body. It also helps to release tension.

2. The practice of Mindful Breathing technique is about focusing on breath taking deep breaths and exhaling at a slow pace.

3. Progressive Muscle Relaxation method involves stretching and relaxing every muscle group of the body to promote relaxation while decreasing tension.

4. The practice is about sending kind and loving thoughts to self and to others, which promotes the relaxation process and decreasing stress.

If you're struggling to insomnia, adding the practice of mindfulness and meditation in your day-to-day routine is beneficial in improving sleeping quality and quantity. Also, it is important to focus on healthy sleep practices by making a bedtime routine that is relaxing and ensuring a regular routine for your sleep.

Mindfulness and Meditation for Pain Management

Chronic pain is an illness that is debilitating and affects millions of people around the world. Conventional medical therapies including medications, as well as surgical procedures, provide short-term relief, but they often come with unwanted adverse consequences. The good news is that mindfulness and meditation offer a non-invasive, efficient method of managing discomfort.

Mindfulness refers to the act of remaining present with the present moment with no judgment or distraction. It is a practice which helps to cultivate mindfulness through calming the mind and raising awareness. These two practices are able to reduce the severity of physical pain as well as the emotional pain that goes from it.

Here are a few ways to integrate mindfulness and meditation into your daily pain management regimen:

1. Begin with breathing awareness Start by lying down or sitting in a comfortable place and pay awareness to your breathing. Concentrate on the feeling of air flowing in the body and then out. If you find your mind wandering to other places, slowly bring it back to the breath.

2. Body scan meditation: This method involves continuously focusing on every aspect of your body from head to toe while bringing attention to the sensations that you experience. Begin with your head, and gradually move towards your feet. If you feel any discomfort or pain, you should create a feeling of acceptance and interest to the situation, instead of judgment or resistance.

3. The practice of loving-kindness meditation is about sending love and compassion to your self and other people. Beginning by channeling these feelings towards yourself first, and then friends, family members and finally all beings. It can

ease emotions of anger, resentment and negative feelings that create more stress.

4. Moving meditation: Tai chi, yoga and qigong are just a few exercises that combine meditation and mindfulness. These exercises can reduce stiffness and pain, in addition to increasing the flexibility and strength.

5. Guided imagery: This method involves picturing a serene or healing landscape for example, an ocean or forest as well as focusing on the feelings that you feel. It can alleviate stress and improve relaxation. This can aid in reducing pain.

It is important to keep in mind that meditation and mindfulness do not replace medical care, but instead as a supplement to it. If you're experiencing persistent discomfort, you should talk to your doctor to figure out the most effective method of treatment that is suitable for your needs. Incorporating the practice of mindfulness and meditation in your routine for pain management is a great method to ease discomfort and enhance your general health.

Chapter 18: Mindfulness And Meditation For Better Relationships

The practice of mindfulness and meditation has an impact that is significant in our interactions with people. Being present and present in our interactions others, we can enhance relationships, improve communication, and develop greater understanding and empathy. Below are a few examples of how meditation and mindfulness can enhance relationships with others:

1. Increased communication: Mindfulness assists to improve our listening skills and become more aware of the feelings and needs of people around us. As we develop mindfulness it helps us take a step back and listen to what people are saying with no judgment or distraction. This helps us to better communicate and prevent misunderstandings.

2. Greater compassion and empathy Mindfulness helps us build an increased

sense of empathy and compassion towards the other. As we engage in mindfulness and meditation, we are more conscious of our emotions and thoughts that help us to understand and be more in tune with the feelings of other people. This may lead to more empathy and compassion within our relationships.

3. More intimate connections: Mindfulness may aid in developing deeper connections to others through making us fully active and involved with our relationships. Through mindfulness practice it helps us get rid of distractions, and to be completely present with those around us. This helps us build deeper and more authentic relationships to others.

4. Reducing conflict: Mindfulness may assist us in decreasing conflict within our relationships because it allows us to be more mindful of our emotions and thoughts, as well as to interact with others by expressing more compassion and

understanding. If we are mindful and meditation, we are less sensitive and more responsive and can assist in reducing conflict and settle differences.

5. Increased awareness of self: Mindfulness helps us to become more self-aware and enhance our interactions with other people. If we are mindful and meditation, we are more conscious of our personal feelings, beliefs and triggers. This helps us to avoid imposing your own problems onto the other person and help create positive relationships.

All in all, mindfulness and meditation can be effective tools for strengthening our connections with other people. Through cultivating awareness, compassion as well as presence, we will be able to strengthen our relationships and build better relationships across every aspect of our life.

www.ingramcontent.com/pod-product-compliance
Lightning Source LLC
Chambersburg PA
CBHW071444080526
44587CB00014B/1980